Humanizing Health Care

Creating Cultures of Compassion
With Nonviolent Communication

Melanie Sears, RN, MBA

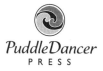

PuddleDancer
P R E S S

2240 Encinitas Blvd., Ste. D-911, Encinitas, CA 92024
email@PuddleDancer.com • www.PuddleDancer.com

For additional information:
Center for Nonviolent Communication
5600-A San Francisco Rd., NE, Albuquerque, NM 87109
Ph: 505-244-4041 • Fax: 505-247-0414 • Email: cnvc@cnvc.org • Website: www.cnvc.org

Humanizing Health Care
Creating Cultures of Compassion With Nonviolent Communication

PuddleDancer Press, Permissions Dept.
2240 Encinitas Blvd., Ste. D-911, Encinitas, CA 92024
Tel: 1-858-759-6963 Fax: 1-858-759-6967
www.NonviolentCommunication.com Email@PuddleDancer.com

Ordering Information
Please contact Independent Publishers Group,
Tel: 312-337-0747; Fax: 312-337-5985; Email: frontdesk@ipgbook.com
or visit www.IPGbook.com for other contact information and details
about ordering online

Author: Melanie Sears

Editor: Sara Saltee

Cover and Interior Design: Lightbourne, Inc., www.lightbourne.com

Indexer: Phyllis Linn, Indexpress

Cover Source Photographs: www.gettyimages.com

Manufactured in the United States of America

1st Printing, August 2010

10 9 8 7 6 5 4 3 2 1

978-1-892005-26-7

What People Are Saying About *Humanizing Health Care*:

"When health care providers know how to communicate clearly about human needs and the emotions that signal them, the entire heath care terrain changes. Hearts open ... and we can all give and receive the best possible health care. Here's my advice. Read and use this book. Its message is life-saving."

—CHRISTIANE NORTHRUP, MD, OB/GYN physician, and author of the *New York Times* bestsellers: *Women's Bodies, Women's Wisdom* and *The Wisdom of Menopause*

"*Humanizing Health Care* is beautifully designed and cogently addresses better communication skills in a straightforward, practical manner. The author discusses psychiatric ward settings for many of her communication examples, but the communication techniques she explains can be used anywhere to improve relations and to more empathically connect with others, be they patients, clients, students, or friends and family. A lovely book."

—PETER R. BREGGIN, MD, author, *Medication Madness, Heart of Being Helpful*, and *Toxic Psychiatry*

"Finally, a book that addresses the need to change our delivery of health care—turn the focus from diagnoses, labels, and judgments into possibilities of health and healing through compassion, caring, and connection."

—SYLVIA HASKVITZ, MA, RD, author, *Eat by Choice, Not by Habit*, and CNVC Certified Trainer

"*Humanizing Health Care* is a valuable resource for all care providers and consumers who are interested in being partners in the recovery process. This book shares practical skills required for use in creating a trauma informed and trauma sensitive environment."

—DONNA RIEMER, RN, PMHN-BC, Certified Traumatologist

"In *Humanizing Health Care*, Melanie Sears provides an invitation for those who lead and work in health care environments to revolutionize the way we provide health care. She provides the tools that will help create the kind of environments that truly provide the safety, the compassion, and the efficiency that our health care systems so desperately need. I dream of working in an environment that has adopted these tools."

—JOAN KELLY, LICSW, GMHS, MT-BC

"As a patient in a psychiatric hospital and a recipient of Mel's empathy skills which she outlines with such clarity in this book, I was able to heal emotionally both from my original wounding and the trauma of being hospitalized. Having a witness to my intense feelings helped me gradually find trust in myself again."

—JOANNE LANE, mother, civil engineer,
and survivor of mental diagnosis

"*Humanizing Health Care* is a call from the heart to transform our health care system into a system that cares about people's health and about the health of the people who work in it. As Melanie articulately and insightfully shows, the two are inseparable. *Humanizing Health Care* teaches honesty without fear, responsibility without blame, and power without exploitation."

—GABOR MATÉ, MD, author of *When The Body Says No:*
Understanding The Stress-Disease Connection

Contents

Preface

Why I wrote this book

I wrote this book because I have seen such suffering among both patients and staff in every health care facility where I have worked. When my own personal journey of healing brought me in touch with Nonviolent Communication (NVC), I knew I had found a set of tools with tremendous potential to put an end to that suffering. As a health care professional, I continue to feel moved by the possibilities of healing the organizations we count on to heal us.

In our current systems, patients suffer because when they are the most vulnerable, the care they receive in hospitals is often mechanical and less than compassionate. All the focus is on a patient's illness and none is on their emotional needs. And more troubling yet is the way our hospitals are organized around the utterly false premise that our physical and emotional selves are two completely separate systems. When we act as if we can treat one without acknowledging the other, the results are damaging and sometimes even catastrophic.

Staff suffer, too, because they work in environments where the lighting is artificial, the noise level is constant, the work hours long, the staffing short, and emergencies involving people's lives are routine. In the midst of such fundamentally stressful environments, staff-to-staff interactions are often hostile and defensive. In settings where teamwork is necessary to deliver quality care and save lives, interpersonal conflicts and closed communication are more often the rule. Most of all, staff suffer because their highest purpose and most compassionate impulses to care and heal are diminished and corrupted by organizations that reinforce artificial power hierarchies and systematically devalue the emotional lives of everyone involved.

I hope that by sharing the tools that were instrumental to me in my own healing journey I can contribute to a more peaceful world and a more compassionate health care system. I am confident that these tools can create systems that serve humanity better by fostering connections rather than violence.

I believe this book will be useful to administrators committed to better patient outcomes, less staff burnout, and better staff relationships. I hope it will also serve the wonderful health care professionals who need to feel understood for their experiences. And, I believe this book will also be healing for patients who have utilized health care and haven't been able to articulate why and how their needs were not met.

Throughout this book, I share stories of specific challenges and solutions I've encountered in my work as a nurse on an involuntary psychiatric unit, and I use these to illustrate how important NVC could be to the health care industry. My belief is that if NVC can create harmony and peace in the emotionally charged environment of a psych unit, there are no limits to how effective it can be in all areas of the hospital.

There are simply no known physical or mental illnesses that cannot be better treated with compassion than without. And, when hospital staff are supported in expressing their natural compassion, speaking the truth, and articulating feelings and needs, the quality of care will—and does—skyrocket. We have it in our power to end the suffering that is so endemic to our health care organizations. What are we waiting for?

Acknowledgments

I want to thank Dr. Marshall Rosenberg for creating the process of Nonviolent Communication (NVC). By using tools of NVC, I've been able to act more in harmony with my inner values rather than from my conditioning. I've become aware of the violence in my heritage and have learned more compassionate ways to interact with myself and others. The tools have enriched my work as a nurse and have enabled me to understand why, for so many people, it is often emotionally painful to work in the health care system.

I discovered the real power of NVC through working on my own issues in groups where people opened their hearts to me and met me with empathy and honesty. I am grateful for the healing experienced and thank all who gave me this gift.

Thanks also to all who have helped me edit this book: Matt Harris, Michael Smith, Joanne Lane, Jocelyn Brown, Elizabeth Burton, and Jen Witsoe.

It is with much gratitude and admiration that I thank Sara Saltee for reorganizing and editing this second edition. Her skill in writing and editing made this book a lot more fun to read.

Chapter 1

A Crisis in Health Care

By many indications, all is not well in the emotional lives of health care workers. Studies show that the suicide rate for male doctors is about 1.4 times the general population, and female doctors commit suicide more than twice as often as women in the general population.[1] Health care practitioners and technicians have a depression rate of 9.6 percent per year. This is 2.6 percent higher than the average for full-time workers.[2] Why are doctors and health care workers so unhappy?

A 1996 Lancet study indicated that doctors and other health care workers commonly struggle with emotional exhaustion, depersonalization (treating people in an impersonal, unfeeling way), low estimation of personal accomplishment, work overload, and poor management and resources. Dealing with the suffering of patients and their distressed, angry, or blaming relatives on a daily basis is extremely taxing.

The doctors in the Lancet study reported their primary sources of job satisfaction were good relationships with patients, relatives, and staff, and having professional status and esteem. They said being understood by management contributed to their happiness, as did enjoying a high degree of autonomy, and performing a variety of tasks.

Significantly, only 45 percent of the doctors in the study thought they had received adequate training in communication skills, while all believed they had received adequate training in the treatment of disease and management of symptoms. As the report reaffirms, "The mental health of (doctors) may nevertheless be protected by maintaining or enhancing their job satisfaction…through giving them autonomy and variety in their work, as well as providing effective training in communication and management skills."[3]

It seems that at least some of the missing pieces in the wellness of health care professionals relate to the personal, human dimensions of their work rather than the technical dimensions: less than half feel adequately prepared to communicate effectively with others, which means less than half feel skilled at connecting in meaningful and effective ways with the people around them. Doctors are also terrified of giving empathy to a patient for fear that it will take too much time. That absence of meaningful connection is surely a contributor to the kind of alienation and depression that underlies the grim suicide statistics.

Health care institutions also feel the costs of these missing pieces. Low job satisfaction and high turnover are extraordinarily costly for hospitals, which shoulder an average cost of $60,000 for every employee turnover. No wonder many hospitals are looking for ways to increase retention and lower recruitment costs!

Some Hopeful Interventions

The evidence shows that health care institutions can successfully reduce retention and recruitment costs by millions of dollars by improving employee satisfaction, and that better communication is a key success factor. In particular, a communication model called Nonviolent Communication (NVC) has been implemented in several health care settings, with powerful results. Some examples include:

- Mercy Hospital in Baltimore implemented NVC into several high-volume outpatient departments. They were so excited with the results that they hired a full-time NVC trainer to train the hospital's entire management team and work force. Since doing this, they have found statistically significant improvement in patient satisfaction, reductions in employee turnover, and improved worker performance.

- Carla Corwith, RN-BA, MBA, and Donna Riemer, RN-BC, Certified Traumatologist, developed a program that included NVC onto the medium security forensic unit at Mendota Mental Health Institute in Wisconsin. Because of this, Seclusion and Restraints (S/R) incidents were reduced from 33 in 2003 to 6 in 2006. S/R hours were reduced from 92.57 hours in 2003 to 6.4 hours in 2006. Time loss from work due to serious staff injuries was reduced from several months to zero. The need for 1:1 staffing—costing tens of thousands of dollars each year—was eliminated.

IMPACT OF NVC ON THE FORENSIC UNIT OF MENDOTA MENTAL HEALTH INSTITUTE		
	2003 (before NVC)	2006 (after NVC)
Seclusion and Restraints incidents	33	6
Seclusion and Restraint hours	92.57	6.4
Time loss due to staff injuries	Several months lost	0
1:1 staffing costs	>$10,000 per year	$0

- In 2008, Donna Riemer went on to develop a similar program that included NVC and integrated it onto the maximum security forensic unit at Mendota, the final stop for the most violent forensic and civil patients in the state of Wisconsin. The results of this strategy were astounding. Staff and patients became partners in recovery. Patients learned how to empathize with staff and staff learned the same. Everyone attended NVC classes every week, and the NVC tools were used daily among staff and patients. The results were a drastic decrease in violence and a change from a violent culture to one of healing. Statistically, there was a 55 percent reduction in the use of the Emergency Intervention Team. This team is called to subdue patients who are acting in violent and destructive ways. The unit has now become safe for both patients and staff.

So, what is NVC? And why is it so effective in improving patient and staff satisfaction, reducing the costs of providing care, and creating cultures of healing?

Notes: _____

1. Dr. Eva S. Schernhammer, M.D., D.P.H. and Graham A Colditz, M.D., D.P.H., "Suicide Rates Among Physicians: A Quantitative and Gender Assessment (Meta-Analysis)," *The American Journal of Psychiatry,* 161:2295-2302 December 2004.
   www.ajp.psychiatryonline.org/cgi/content/full/161/12/2295
2. "Depression Among Adults Employed Full-time by Occupational Category," Office of Applied Studies in the U.S. Department of Health and Human Services.
   www.oas.samhsa.gov/2k7/depression/occupation.cfm
3. Ramirez AJ, Graham J, Richards MA, Cull A, Gregory WM, "Mental Health of Hospital Consultants: The Effects of Stress and Satisfaction at Work," *The Lancet*, Volume 347, Issue 9003, pp. 724–28, March 16, 1996.
   www.thelancet.com/journals/lancet/article/PIIS0140-6736(96)90077-X/abstract

Chapter 2

Understanding Nonviolent Communication

What Is Nonviolent Communication?

Nonviolent Communication (NVC) is a philosophy, a leadership technique, and a system of communication that empowers individuals to achieve greater empathy for others by developing their own sense of their feelings and needs. NVC can be used to heal emotional wounds, develop emotional intelligence, resolve conflicts, and create win-win solutions. It can be used in all relationships: at work, as a parent, as a partner, as a friend. It enhances one's sense of security so that other voices can be heard which opens up communication and creates understanding. Applying the principles and practices of NVC enables people to take control of their lives and to maintain integrity consistent with their deepest values.

Dr. Marshall Rosenberg, founder and director of educational services for the Center for Nonviolent Communication, developed the NVC model in the early 1960s. In search of ways to support peaceful desegregation of schools and other institutions, he began to study the practices of good communicators. His studies culminated in a four-step model of communication that emphasizes honesty, empathy, and awareness of the power of words to shape perceptions of reality. Today,

Dr. Rosenberg travels all around the world teaching this process, resolving conflicts in war-torn countries, and helping people live peaceful, joyful lives by shifting their communication.[1]

As he studied the question, "What keeps us connected to our naturally compassionate nature?'" Dr. Rosenberg began to understand that our patterns of communication literally create the world that we experience. The messages you deliver to yourself in your own head and the messages you deliver to the people you live and work with powerfully shape your perception and your relationships. In a workplace, these communication practices combine to create the culture you share.

When you act out destructive communication patterns without an awareness of doing so, you unwittingly become co-creators of dehumanizing cultures that never acknowledge or address the real needs of the people involved. But, when you become conscious of your communication patterns and develop choice in how you think and react, then you literally change the world in which you live. When you connect the words you use with your own honest feelings and needs and use them to make clear requests of others, you create meaningful connections with others and with yourself and create effective and lasting change. By implementing NVC, health care institutions can become life-serving environments that better meet the needs of both employees and patients.

How Does NVC Work?

NVC breaks down communications into four steps: Observations, Feelings, Needs, and Requests. Your habitual language often mixes these steps together and leaves out the feelings and the needs. In society in general, and certainly in workplaces, you don't discuss your feelings and needs, instead focusing your attention outward in patterns like: judging, analyzing, blaming, labeling, criticizing, and complimenting. All of these communication activities are oriented toward an outward focus of attention instead of an inward one. Learning to express yourself using NVC shifts your focus inward, allowing honest expression, healing, and growth.

Step One: Observations

The first step in creating clear communication is to be able to state clear observations without mixing in evaluations. Observations are things a video camera can pick up. They contain the observable facts. When the observations are mixed in with feelings, evaluations or judgments are created.

For example: "You are obviously too lazy to take out the garbage." is a statement that clearly combines an observation with an evaluation. By contrast, "I see you did not take out the garbage today," is an observation.

Step Two: Feelings

The second step is to express "Feelings" clearly without blaming or analyzing others. Many people find this step challenging, because they don't have a "feeling vocabulary." Words that mix feelings with analysis or other forms of evaluations are used far more commonly than "feeling words."

Some examples of common words that mix feelings and evaluation are: *used, abused, betrayed, attacked, manipulated, neglected, rejected,* and *threatened.* These words are more about analyzing what someone else is doing wrong than in expressing feelings. When you express yourself using these words, it will often stimulate a defensive reaction in others.

Feeling words, such as *hurt, scared, sad, excited, happy, irritated, confused,* and *surprised* will create connections instead of defensive reactions.

Step Three: Needs

The third step of the NVC process is "Needs." When someone speaks, they're meeting a need. When someone punches another in the nose, they're expressing a need. Uncovering what need the person is expressing allows you to connect with this individual and begins to unlock unconscious motives and moves the person toward self-awareness.

Often when you express yourself, you are not aware of what needs you are trying to express. One reason for this is that you have grown up in a society that has an outward focus instead of an inward focus, and you have become disconnected from your needs. Many of you have been punished for expressing your needs. You have been told that you are selfish or inconsiderate when you asked for what you wanted. In order to understand others' needs, it is important to become aware of your own.

Similarly, you don't often seek to understand the needs that others are expressing through their communication. By focusing your awareness on people's needs instead of judging them for speaking or acting in ways that you don't enjoy, you see the truth of who they are. This allows you to notice that they are not very different from you.

Being out of touch with your own needs and those of others creates disharmony and prevents conflicts from being resolved. When you express your needs and hear others' needs, you discover your common humanity. Barriers between you dissolve. Conflicts are resolved when both parties can hear each other's needs. Trying to solve problems or conflicts before getting clear on what the needs are will create disharmony and negative feelings.

There are many different needs that all people have in common. Manfred Max-Neef, the Chilean economist and environmentalist, has organized them into the following nine categories: Sustenance, protection, affection, understanding, participation, leisure, creation, identity, freedom.[2]

Step Four: Requests

The fourth step is the "request.'" Becoming conscious of what you want back from others when you speak creates safety and self-responsibility. It also improves efficiency. Requests can also be thought of as the strategy for meeting the need. I often hear people use many words when they speak, and they repeat what they are saying. They are not clear what need they are meeting by speaking and what they want back from the person they are speaking to. If they were aware that they needed empathy (for example), then they could ask for that directly and the connection would likely be more satisfying for everyone involved.

There are two types of requests: 1) the Connecting Request and 2) the Solution Request. The first one creates connection between you and others. An example of that request may sound like, "How do you feel about what I just said?" The second request creates a solution to a problem. It could sound like, "Would you be willing to take out the trash?" Requests are action-oriented and "doable" in the present moment.

Putting It All Together

By separating communications into these four steps, you become smarter about how you get your needs met. When you begin to habitually:

- Separate observations from evaluations,
- Identify and express your feelings,
- Determine and express the needs that drive your feelings, and
- Make clear requests using positive action language,

you take responsibility and control of your own experience in a striking new way.

Beyond the Four Steps

The four steps—observations, feelings, needs, and requests—are the cornerstones of the practice of NVC. To fully understand NVC, however, you must also take a look at four principles from which these practices arise:

1. Each of you is responsible for choosing your reactions to people and events;
2. Each of you is also responsible for your own feelings;
3. Your needs are a gift, not a burden, to others;
4. The experience of empathy is at the heart of effective communication.

Principle 1: Each of you is responsible for choosing your reactions to people and events.

I'm sure you have heard the expression, "you create your own reality." This belief may feel debatable during the course of a day when you are affected by people and situations that you seemingly have no control over.

You may not be able to control people and events that you encounter, but you can control how you react to them. When Nelson Mandela was in prison, he chose how he wanted to react to the violent treatment. Instead of being angry and filling himself with hate, he acted compassionately, maintained his dignity, and gained the respect of his guards and fellow prisoners.

Anyone can choose how they want to react to situations and the language you choose can help you stay connected to your inner intentions. Language contains a panoply of philosophies and values. By choosing your style of language, you change the way you react to situations—and often the strategies you use to meet your needs. The language you choose can create cooperation and empowerment for others, or it can create resistance and hostility. The language choices you make will determine the results you get.

Principle 2: Each of you is also responsible for your own feelings.

There are some myths around feelings that need to be cleared up before communications can flow. One of these is that "other people cause your feelings." When you think about this myth logically, it is easy to see that other people don't cause your feelings. Other people can stimulate your feelings, but your feelings are caused by your needs. If your needs are being met, you have positive feelings. If your needs are not being met, you have negative feelings.

Consider the example when someone says, "No." If it is your two-year-old saying, "No," you may feel frustrated because you want to get to work on time. If it is your boss who says, "No," you may feel hurt because you want recognition for your ideas. If it is a friend who said, "No," you may feel happy because you are glad your friend feels safe enough with you to express her truth.

The key insight here is that *it is not the other person but your inner needs that create your feelings.* And the inverse is also true: You do not cause feelings in others. Their feelings are expressions of their own internal experience.

Often you learn that it is OK to have certain positive feelings but that you are judged if you have negative feelings. People judge you because they don't know how to respond to feelings in other ways. Also, hearing feelings will often trigger unresolved issues in others. You are taught to take responsibility for other people's feelings, so it is frightening to express feelings or to hear another's feelings.

From the perspective of the NVC model, feelings are neither good nor bad; they are simply expressions of the internal experience. When you realize that you don't cause other people's feelings, you can begin to be honest about your own feelings and needs. If you express your truth and someone has a defensive reaction to what you say, you know that his or her reaction is about him or her and not about you. You quit taking things personally.

Principle 3: Your needs are a gift, not a burden, to others.

Most of you grew up with two big myths about your own needs—you were taught that your needs are a burden to others, and that if someone really cares for you, they will intuit what you need and give it to you without your having to ask. This combination of beliefs creates distorted and dishonest communication patterns.

Believing that your needs are a burden, you are afraid and ashamed to ask for what you want. You believe you are expressing your compassion for others by "sparing them" the truth of your needs.

Believing that others should know your needs without your having to speak of them, you feel resentful asking for what you want because you interpret the other person as not caring. (If they cared, then you wouldn't have had to ask.)

In order to make clear requests, it is necessary to change your underlying belief system. When you change your belief from "your needs are a burden" to "your needs are a gift" to others, you can then be reassured that it is OK to ask for what you want. When you receive a "No" back from your request, you can empathize instead of punishing the responding person.

You also need to change your belief that people "should" give you what you want without your having to ask. It would make it easier for you to make requests and receive "No" in a compassionate way if you understand that caring is about communicating your feelings and needs directly, receiving others' feelings and needs, and not about reading minds.

Principle 4: The experience of empathy is at the heart of constructive communication.

To have empathy for someone is to clearly understand what feelings and needs they are communicating (either verbally or nonverbally) and to have compassion for them. This requires you to shed all judgments and preconceived ideas and listen with your whole being, not merely with your ears.

In other words, empathy requires being present in the moment and open to the process that is unfolding. Presence creates a sense of freedom in the person to whom you are listening and allows them to touch deeper levels of themselves. The quality of your presence might seem like an intangible concept, but people can instantly sense whether you are present or not, and your presence has the power to create the environment in which they experience themselves.

Receiving unconditional acceptance through empathy allows others to accept themselves, as illustrated in the following letter I received from a patient: "Thanks for being so likeable and so affirming. Seeing myself through your eyes gave me the freedom to judge myself less and love myself a little more." The quality of my compassionate presence created the space within which this patient could alter her own experience of herself.

What's the difference between empathy and active listening? Active listening is focused more on mentally understanding what someone is saying. It does not necessarily involve listening and expressing true empathy. For example, therapists often think they are being empathic when they listen to people's words carefully in order to connect them to preexisting theories or diagnostic categories. Rather than hearing the feelings and needs under the patient's words, the therapist in this case is actually listening for cues and clues as to which box or frame the patient best fits within. The therapist's emphasis is on studying a person instead of being with them.

The word *empathy* is also often confused with sympathy. Sympathy is more akin to pity. It occurs when one person feels sorry for another. Empathy, on the other hand, occurs between equals where one heart is open to another's. When I use the word *empathy* in this book, I am referring to a specific consciousness of connection and a specific technology. Empathy used in this sense is akin to the state of presence that is practiced by some evolved spiritual leaders. You don't need to be an evolved spiritual leader though to use the tools of empathy. Guessing what people may be feeling and needing is about connecting with the humanity in yourself and in others. Focusing your attention on someone's feelings and needs creates a space for that person to begin inner exploration. It doesn't matter if you accurately guess the feelings and needs being expressed. A correct guess or an incorrect guess will help bring a person closer to their own inner experience. Being empathic involves focusing on the feelings and needs being expressed in each and every second.

Being empathic in this way involves getting yourself out of the way. What the person is expressing is not about you. If you take it personally, give advice, or tell your own story in response to what the person is saying, then you are blocking communication. In fact, though most of you believe that you are empathic people, often the language you use to express your empathy sounds judgmental or analytical. When you advise, console, educate, interrogate, sympathize, analyze, explain, or correct, you are not empathizing. The words used in empathy express feelings and needs. Because you all share feelings and needs in common, the language of feelings and needs is empowering and creates a human bond between people. Being heard clearly for your feelings and needs with no judgments, labels, or analysis frees the heart to open and express whatever is inside.

Let's work through an example of how empathic communication sounds different from the languages of judgment, sympathy, etc. Let's assume you are a staff member and a patient asks you the provocative question: *"What did I do wrong to be placed in this hellhole?"* Here is a range of possible response styles:

Questioning: "What do you think you did?"

Analysis: "You are acting like a 'borderline.'"

Active listening: "I hear you asking what you did wrong to be placed in this hellhole."

Advising: "You need to calm down and take your medications."

Correcting: "This is not a hellhole, it's a Psychiatric Unit."

Consoling: "You didn't do anything wrong. You'll feel better soon."

Educating: "This is a chance for you to work on your issues."

Empathizing: "Are you feeling angry and do you need information about why you are here?"

Interestingly, the empathizing response is the least likely to create a defensive reaction. However, it is important to know that when you hear someone with empathy, the feelings of the person expressing may initially get more intense. As you continue to empathize with them, though, there will be a calming effect. People who are unsure of their empathy skills often grow frightened when they see this escalation of feelings and then resort to power over tactics. If you stay calm and continue to focus your attention on the feelings and needs being expressed, you will find that a connection is created and trust is established.

What words express feelings? This is trickier than you might think because some words that are commonly thought of as "feeling words" actually express thoughts. These words actually express an analysis of what someone is doing to you and by being attached to thinking in these terms one can stay stuck in a state of being a victim. When you use these "thought" words (such as abused, abandoned, attacked, betrayed, bullied, cheated, diminished, intimidated, manipulated, misunderstood, neglected, pressured, provoked, put down, rejected, threatened, unwanted, used, etc.) to reflect back your understanding of what someone is saying, it will often reinforce their own powerlessness.

When you give empathy to someone who uses these "thought" words, you look underneath them to the feelings and needs being expressed. In essence, you learn how to translate thoughts into feelings and needs. For example, a person who says, "He used me," may be feeling hurt and may need understanding for her distress. Accurately expressing empathy would sound like: "Are you feeling hurt and need understanding for your distress?" You would not say, "Are you feeling used?" as this would reinforce the existing perception of powerlessness.

Which words express needs? It is common to confuse words that express needs with words that express strategies. Needs are the universal, underlying sources of life energy shared by all human beings in all times and all cultures. For instance, everyone has a need for security but in different cultures, this security need is met through very different strategies. In some cultures, people stockpile dollars in the bank in order to meet needs for security, while in tribal cultures the same need for security may be met through accumulation of livestock. Some people get their need for security met by belonging to an extended family, others find it by doing meaningful work. There are many different strategies to meet the same need.

Communication opens when the focus is on needs and can become entangled when the focus is on strategies. You may not condone a person's strategies, but by connecting with their needs, it is possible to have compassion for him or her. Also, by teasing the need apart from all the strategies you are using to try to meet the need, you can often come to see why your strategies aren't working well, and you can have greater insight into the strategies that are more congruent with your core needs.

Not only can staff support patients by offering empathy but they can also support one another. When employees feel discouraged or upset over an interaction, others can offer them empathy. When interpersonal conflicts arise, it is essential to have empathy skills in order to create connection and reach win-win solutions. When someone is angry, empathy can diffuse his or her anger and heal the problem.

Empathy is needed to build successful teams and for creating community.

It is critical, however, to know that before you can be empathic toward others, you must first be clear and connected with yourself. You can be present to others to the extent that you have done your own inner healing work. Being unable to empathize with someone is an indication that some issue or judgment you have is in the way. By focusing your attention inward toward your own feelings and needs, you can find out what is in the way of being present to others. Using the tools of NVC, you can become clearer and more connected with yourself and with others. The degree of empathy you have for yourself is the degree that you will be able to empathize with others.

Shifting Consciousness

Once you begin to work with these four core concepts of NVC:
- Each of you is responsible for choosing your reactions to people and events;
- Each of you is also responsible for your own feelings;
- Your needs are a gift, not a burden, to others;
- The experience of empathy is at the heart of constructive communication;

you set in motion a shift in consciousness that can powerfully alter your relationship to yourself and others. By shifting your consciousness and communication from outward to inward, and by paying attention to what is going on inside yourself and others, the world you live in literally begins to change.

Think about that: the world you live in literally begins to change as you shift your perceptions and use new language. Of course, I'm writing this book because I believe that this consciousness shift is a change for the better, and this book is full of stories of the transformational results that occur once individuals and whole organizations begin to practice empathy for feelings and needs. I hope you'll come to see how meeting human emotional needs can be more effective than medication, how health care staff members could work less hard and have better results, and how expressing respect for the human beings around you is a cornerstone of effective partnership cultures.

However, as you begin to test for yourself the consciousness shift of NVC, I also want you to be aware that people who occupy a different perceptual framework will have a very difficult time making sense of what is going on in the practice of NVC. People very literally cannot see what they are not prepared to see, so the effects of NVC often seem magical or mysterious or just invisible to people who are not grounded in the concepts and practices of NVC.

Philosopher Arthur Schopenhauer said: "All truth passes through three stages. First, it is ridiculed. Second, it is violently opposed. Third, it is accepted as being self-evident."[3] If you think of NVC as a system for perceiving truth in a new way, it makes sense to expect that people who are not seeing the world through the NVC lens will very often ridicule it, oppose it, or go to great lengths to develop alternative explanations for the effects that NVC has on human relationships. These natural processes humans use to distance themselves from what they don't yet understand is important to be aware of as you seek to embed NVC principles into your life as an individual or into the culture of your organization.

Let me offer an example: One evening, in the psychiatric medicine unit, I was caring for a forty-year-old woman, Ann, who weighed three hundred fifty pounds. Her weight is relevant because several times a day—at least once during every shift—she would lie on the floor and scream and cuss out the staff. This caused a significant problem for staff. Because they were unable to lift her up by themselves, they had to call the lift team each time they wanted to get her off of the floor, and they worried that if they called the lift team every time Ann was on the floor that her behavior would be reinforced. So, they adopted a strategy of ignoring Ann's outbursts as best they could.

The evening I took care of Ann, however, she did not lie on the floor nor did she scream and yell. When the staff noticed that she had acted differently than usual, they reached first for an explanation that fit within their existing belief system, and they concluded that "the meds must be kicking in." Of course, this was a logical conclusion to reach, within a perceptual framework in which medications are the privileged route to behavior change.

But this time that wasn't an accurate explanation. It wasn't medication at all that changed Ann's behavior, it was the way I talked with and connected with her. I entered Ann's room mindful of the NVC core concepts that all human beings are always trying to meet their needs and that no matter how violent the behavior, it is possible to connect to a person's heart through empathic communication. I encouraged Ann to express her feelings and I reflected back her unconscious needs. Because Ann felt nurtured and heard, she did not try and get her needs met by lying on the floor. Her needs for understanding and attention were met by what I was doing so she "magically" didn't have to act out.

The rest of the staff were very surprised that I was having such an "easy shift" since caring for this patient was usually quite challenging. When I suggested that perhaps it was not the meds that were making the difference but the way I was working with the patient, staff members refused to believe it. Since they had not experienced the paradigm of NVC and the power of empathy and compassion themselves, they literally could not see it in action.

This example reminds you why it is so important to think about adopting NVC at the organizational level. Clearly, any one individual using NVC practices can do great things and can become a force for healing in themselves and those whose lives they touch. But imagine the potential impact when a whole organizational system works together within a shared communication framework!

Suddenly, instead of evaluating and judging others, you find yourself listening to them because you care about who they really are. By listening instead of judging, you discover that people are compassionate. They want to help others and to contribute to the workplace and to society. They want to experience security, respect, love, understanding, and more—just as you do.

When you understand this ("understand" with your hearts as well as your heads), you naturally come to see, to "believe," that people are compassionate. When an organization understands this, it's much more likely to create systems that meet people's needs. But it's important to stress that this understanding needs to come from within—from the heart. Merely changing the externals will fail until underlying principles, myths, and ways of thinking change.

Now that you have a fuller understanding of the four steps of the NVC process and some of the core concepts of NVC, let's begin to look at how NVC can help to shift your health care organizations from domination systems to partnership systems that meet the needs of staff and patients alike.

Notes: _____

1. Rosenberg, Marshall, *Nonviolent Communication: A Language of Life*, second edition, (Encinitas, California: PuddleDancer Press, 2003). Also see www.NonviolentCommunication.com and www.cnvc.org
2. "Max-Neef on Human Needs and Human-scale Development." www.rainforestinfo.org.au/background/maxneef.htm
3. www.brainyquote.com/quotes/authors/a/arthur_schopenhauer.html

Chapter 3

From Domination to Partnership: The Evolution of Health Care Systems

In almost every type of human system, you can see an evolutionary shift at work. In family life, in business, in international relations, in gender relations, in politics, in education, and, yes, even in health care organizations, a long and powerful tradition of domination-based systems is giving way to a partnership model. This evolutionary shift is not occurring without struggle; change is not simple and it does not happen all at once. But in almost every domain of social relationships, old reliance on rigid hierarchies and "power over" is being challenged by relationships based on mutuality, shared power, and collaboration toward the common good.

Partnership Models at Home

The example of your family relationships offers a clear and vivid example. Within the span of just a few generations, the dominant model of family relationship has shifted from domination to partnership. I remember vividly the experience of childhood in a dominance-oriented family. I got messages such as "Children are to be seen and not heard," "I'll give you something to cry about," and "Do it my way because I said so." These messages are all indicators of a model in which the power dynamics are hierarchical and one-way: parents are all-powerful "experts" and children are relatively powerless and expected to submit to their parents' will.

Contrast this family system model with family relationships of many families today: Parents I work with in my Nonviolent Communication (NVC) business are eager to take a more respectful approach to childrearing than their parents and grandparents did. Those who experienced being raised in a domination model worry that perpetuating that system in their own families will undermine their connection with their children. They are seeking ways to foster loving relationships with children without resorting to power over tactics. My own experience suggests that this is not just a dream.

I used NVC to help guide me in raising my children and I enjoy a much closer relationship with my grown children than my parents have with me. This is because I keep the communication open by listening instead of scolding, by trusting instead of punishing, and by understanding instead of judging. Like me, many parents today invite their children's participation in family choice-making, make more requests and fewer demands, and seek to empower their children by enabling children to exercise their own power of choice-making.

Partnership Models in Business

Consider also the way the domination model has transformed in the business world. The change to partnership systems in business is occurring partially because research has shown that businesses are more profitable when workers are internally motivated. Old strategies of motivating through financial rewards, threats of punishment, or words of praise are only effective in the short term. After a while, workers become suspicious that they are being manipulated and their performance drops off. External motivations, once the industry standard, are now being challenged. The only way that employees can be truly motivated is to be inspired by their job, to have input in designing and organizing their work, and to find meaning and purpose in their contributions. Many businesses have changed from top-down hierarchies to other organizational structures that encourage teamwork and information-sharing. In order to stay competitive, many businesses encourage individual creativity and support employees in developing solutions at every level of the organization, not waiting for answers to be delivered "from above."

What About Health Care?

Those health care organizations that have already begun to transform business as usual through intentional development of partnership-based relationships have improved outcomes for employees, patients, and organizations as a whole, and the practices of Nonviolent Communication can be an important part of that transformation. NVC does more than just support a shift from relationships of domination to human partnerships, it actually *creates* the shift by disarming the language of domination and replacing it with language that humanizes and empowers everyone in the system.

Before going further to explore the ways in which NVC supports and enables partnership systems in health care, however, let's take a closer look at how domination systems really work, and acknowledge the damaging impacts they've historically had on health care institutions, the people who work in them, and the people who seek healing from them. A deeper understanding of the dynamics of domination is an important part of moving toward something better. By accurately naming what is, you can begin to see how change is possible and necessary.

What Is a Domination System?

Domination structures were developed thousands of years ago when our ancestors moved from small-scale gardening to larger-scale farming. Because physical strength was needed to handle plows and other implements of mass food production, physically strong men found themselves increasingly in positions of power, and systems of domination began to evolve. A cultural spiritual shift occurred at this time away from reverence for life and pleasure and toward domination and pain. "In order to maintain rigid rankings of domination, violence and abuse became institutionalized and (as with unprosecuted male violence of both warfare and the war of the sexes) bound up with gender-specific socialization processes."[1]

In domination systems, there are two roles: those who dominate and those who are dominated. Those on top control those below and benefit from their position at the expense of others. Those who are dominated often come to believe that they, too, benefit from the perpetuation of the domination system—after all, "Father Knows Best." The system is held in place through fear and force and through patterns of thinking that polarize complex feelings and experiences into strict categories: Right or Wrong, Good or Bad, Us or Them, Punishment or Reward.

The Downsides of Dominance

Dependency

Let's look again at the example of the family to see the impact of dominance systems. In the family context, you can see how dominance-based parenting perpetuates a sense of dependency and teaches children to blindly obey external authorities. This learned dependency has far-reaching social consequences, too; by socializing people to blindly obey authority figures, you ensure that people lose touch with their own sense of self-responsibility and expect others to fix their problems. People socialized in this way allow others to control decisions that affect them, and then seethe with resentment. Partly they are afraid that if they speak up, they will be punished; and partly they don't know how to express themselves and break the pattern of silence that has been handed down for thousands of years.

Domination system language creates and perpetuates the myth that most people are incapable of rational thought by themselves and need to be told what to think by others who are better educated, more intelligent, or morally superior. This belief system creates profound problems in organizations because people have needs (such as autonomy and respect) that cannot be satisfactorily met with such an underlying belief system.

From a health care standpoint, this attitude expresses itself when instead of taking control of their health and developing a healthy lifestyle, people expect a pill or an operation to fix them. The current heath care system depends on this attitude in order to continue operating as it does now. When a patient is anxious, they take a pill. When someone gets lung disease from smoking, they take multiple medications and are frequently hospitalized. Instead of preventing the disease in the first place or finding ways to soothe and heal emotional issues, this dependency on the heath care system as a whole and the authorities (doctors) who work there feeds the health care system.

Devaluing of Caring and Empathy

Relationships of dominance cannot be sustained unless everyone in the system is socialized to suppress or ignore their true feelings and needs. Both dominators and those who submit to domination are socialized to repress feelings of anger, and to be ashamed of their human needs for empathy, honesty, and care.

Exerting power over others requires human beings to "be tough." This "toughness" allows the dominator to play the power over role, but requires the suppression of the dominator's own needs for human connection based not on status or role, but on recognition of their deepest inner qualities. The dominator's "toughness" is shored up through minimizing and ridiculing the "soft" human needs for connection, recognition, empathy, and care. "To maintain rankings of domination, caring and empathy have to be suppressed and devalued, beginning in families and from there to economics and politics."[2]

Submitting to the power of others who you perceive as "above" you also does violence. As you shape your will to conform to the requests of those in power, you must suppress your own will, and learn to turn a deaf ear to the wisdom within. The wisdom of caring, empathy, and human connection is particularly suspect within domination systems, as are the people who have historically held this wisdom. The devaluation of the caring professions such as nursing is a "function of the cultural devaluation of anything stereotypically associated with women and femininity...and adversely affects all of us."[3]

Health Care: A Legacy of Domination

In health care systems, the slow shift toward partnership has been particularly noticeable during the last twenty years. There are now more women physicians, and Western medicine is beginning to incorporate techniques such as acupuncture, hypnosis, and healing touch into its patient care. Some physicians and nurses are fed up with the dehumanizing way they are treated and are expected to treat patients. They are forming groups such as The Holistic Nurses Association and the Medical Renaissance Group to support one another and to find strategies to change the system.

Health care providers *want* to meet patients' needs; indeed, the survival of the general system of health care depends on this. However, changing external systems without addressing the structures of control and communication that create them will not adequately meet this task until the underlying principles, myths, and ways of thinking change.

Though Western medicine is struggling to evolve away from its roots in domination, and has made real strides in some areas, health care organizations are still permeated with relationships of domination. Doctors are dominant over nurses, and have knowledge about disease that places them in a position of power over patients who are desperate to heal. Nurses seek dominance over one another and their patients, and use their knowledge of disease to try and meet needs for respect and control. Health care organizations themselves dominate their employees through systems of hierarchical communication, structures of reward and punishment, processes that promote control, and rigid status structures that determine perceptions of worth.

As you've seen, a key feature of being socialized within a domination system is that people look to external authority to tell them how to think and feel. For example, let's say the Charge Nurse doesn't like a particular staff member named George. Chances are, the rest of the staff will also act in cold and indifferent ways toward George. However, if the Physician comes along and praises George, other staff members will suddenly act friendlier to him. George's qualities as a person are unchanging, but the perceptions of him shift depending on how he is perceived by people in positions of authority. If George is fully socialized to accept the logic of the domination system he is in, his own self-perception may shift, too; he may feel like a "loser" when he sees himself through the Charge Nurse's eyes and a "winner" when the Physician praises his work. Like the people around him, George may not trust his own inner experience of who he is, relying instead on the people around him to tell him if he's a winner or loser that day.

The ways in which those with higher status determine your perceptions of reality can be difficult to see, because the pattern is so deeply ingrained. Here's another simple example from my own experience in a setting far from a clinic or hospital. I took a painting class and completed an assignment to paint a still life of a collection of fruit. When I brought the painting to class, my fellow art students laughed and criticized my banana. When the teacher saw my painting, he praised the banana. After the teacher made his comments, my peers stopped laughing and told me what a great banana it was! Clearly, their perceptions of reality shifted to match the view of the person with the highest status in the room. The "truth" about my banana shifted before my eyes, and helped me recognize that I'd better learn to find and trust my own inner truth, or I'd be forever at the mercy of the "fruit judges" with the most status on a given day.

How Status-based Systems Suppress Learning

In health care, as in most of society, the treatment you receive is largely dependent on your status and ranking in the domination system, and your status is marked by your title. In health care, an "Attending" is better than a "Resident," a "RN III" is better than a "RN II." The people at the top of the heap are perceived as better than the people below. Respectful treatment is dependent on your title, and both status and titles are tied to perceptions of competence and expertise.

This emphasis on earning respect through expertise creates systems in which not knowing is perceived as failure, and attempts to learn are judged as evidence of incompetence. If you are new to a certain unit or learning about a new area of medicine, you are often judged until you know what you are doing. I experienced this judgment every time I changed jobs to a new field of nursing, and I've seen it happen to others. For example, I recall a time when a new patient was admitted to a psychiatric unit at the beginning of the evening shift. The Attending had left for the day and a Resident was called to admit the patient. The Resident phoned the Attending for some advice—whereupon the Attending turned her car around and returned to the unit. Word spread throughout the unit, "Watch the Resident, she doesn't know what she's doing." Later the Resident shared with me that she was feeling distressed because she'd picked up that she was being called "incompetent." She was confused as to how she could have acted differently considering that she was new to psychiatry and just learning the ropes.

Being judged for making good faith efforts to learn and improve makes people afraid to ask questions or admit they don't know something. Rather than open themselves up to judgments of incompetence, professionals within health care systems frequently "cover up" their lack of understanding and feel enormous pressure to behave dishonestly, acting as if they know more than they do. This system endangers patients because instead of asking questions, people perform procedures without understanding what they're doing. It also creates an environment where being truthful about who you are and what you don't know is dangerous to your reputation and self esteem.

Here's an example of how easily this dynamic of "faking it" to avoid losing status can create negative consequences. Though the story has a happy ending, it is not hard to see how a similar situation in which questions are left unasked for fear of judgment could have terrible consequences. Shortly after graduating from nursing school, I was "floated" to work on Post Partum, where I was instructed to set up a breast pump for a patient. I'd never seen a breast pump before and, when I asked where it was, the nurse said in an angry voice, "It's in the hall." She then turned and walked away. When I sensed how stressed and angry she was, I was hesitant to chase after her and ask for clarification. I saw a machine in the hall and took it into the patient's room. I attached the breast tubing to the machine and turned it on. It seemed to fit together fine and to be working well so I left the room. The next day, a Resident came up to me, laughing, and said, "Who hooked the woman's boob up to Gomco Suction, Melanie?" (A Gomco Suction Machine® is used to put negative pressure on wound drains to keep them draining. It works quite differently than a breast pump.) Thank goodness, there was not a bad outcome for this patient. Since then, I have had to struggle to learn new things, treading lightly, lest I trigger irritation in others by asking questions.

What Does the Language of Domination Sound Like? And How Does It Hinder the Goals of Health Care?

You've seen how the legacy of domination impacts health care organizations by disassociating people from their own perception of truth and by squelching learning. But perhaps the deepest wound of domination is in the way you are habituated to use language. Communication patterns are shaped by belief systems that are perpetuated through language. Language expresses and creates your consciousness in relation to your worldview. As long as you continue to rely on unconscious language patterns that perpetuate old systems, you will be hard pressed to create a shift toward treating patients holistically and compassionately. You must intentionally move away from the old hierarchical and dominating language patterns that minimize people's feelings and needs.

In domination systems, the focus of attention is outward, and the communication patterns of domination reflect this emphasis on controlling and judging the world outside of yourself. Language that blames and threatens, compliments and criticizes, reprimands and rewards, supports "power over" structures common in domination systems. Outwardly focused communication is also rife with evaluations, diagnoses, labels, judgments, and analyses. Since motivation is extrinsic and systems of reward and punishment are widespread, the language in domination systems is full of such words as *"have to," "should," "must,"* and *"deserve."*

The use of domination language, particularly the language of labeling and analyzing others undermines the healing mission of health care environments by deepening and perpetuating a patient's pain. Here's one small example of the negative power of such language. During report on the inpatient unit one evening, I was told that a patient I had been assigned to work with was a "sad sack." This label, of course, implied a judgment: It is not OK to be sad, and it is particularly not OK to not be able to contain and suppress one's sadness "appropriately." After report, the patient met me in the hall crying and asked to speak with me. I gave myself a moment to self-connect before agreeing to meet with her. When I looked inside, I noticed that I had colluded with the person giving report and was myself judging this patient as a "sad sack." This was unlike me because I usually like people who are able to express their feelings. I noticed the pull to get my need met for belonging and acceptance by conforming to the group culture.

How destructive it can be to work in an organization where this domination consciousness is the norm! It is very difficult to stay connected to one's true values when your peers are acting and thinking in a violent way that is supported by the system. After I regained connection with my own compassion, I sat with the patient and gave her empathy for her distress. I listened closely for about ten minutes, reflecting back the feelings and needs I heard her express. When she stopped crying, we started joking and laughing. We both felt an easy connection with each other. This patient had been crying all day trying to get her need met for understanding. Once she felt understood, she stopped crying and started participating in the activities on the unit.

And here's another example of how the words used by health care workers affect patients' behavior. Last night, I heard a nurse tell a patient, "You are taking up too much of my time." This upset the patient, who started crying. For the next two hours, the patient hung around the nurses' station, asking every staff person to help her with some task. It was a busy night and the staff members were stressed so no one wanted to help this patient whom they had labeled, "needy." I stopped what I was doing and went to the patient's room with her to listen to her distress. I gave her empathy and showed caring for her needs. The patient calmed down after this and went to bed. Ten minutes of quality empathy and attention had soothed the patient so she no longer tried to get her needs met in ways that were judged as irritating and needy.

How is it possible that a simple sentence like "You are taking up too much of my time" is actually a form of violence? Why would it stimulate such a painful reaction? Let's look closely at what is happening in that sentence. The first word, *"You,"* is an outward-directed communication that implies blame. With the words "are taking up," the speaker is accusing the listener of being greedy, of having needs that are too big and not appropriate. The words *too much* are unclear and imply a judgment. The sentence as a whole is an outward-directed analysis of what this patient is doing wrong. There is no self-responsibility being expressed in this sentence.

Now, you can empathize and understand that the nurse who expressed herself this way was feeling stressed out. This nurse is very conscientious. It troubles her when she cannot meet her patient's needs. However, she is also human and when the unit is short-staffed, she becomes irritable because she cannot do the kind of job that would give her satisfaction. She was irritated when the patient asked her to do things for her because she wanted to get her work done before the end of the shift. But what was the result of her language? Ironically, the nurse created more of the very thing she didn't want. As soon as she expressed domination over the patient with the phrase *You are taking up too much of my time*, the patient became upset and promptly began to need even more care. The sentence *You are taking up too much of my time* is an example of what happens when blaming judgmental language is used that implies wrongness. This one sentence illustrates several habitual patterns of speech and the consciousness underneath the words that can stimulate pain and violence in others. This patient reacted by crying. Another patient could react by throwing a chair across the room.

So, how might the nurse have used language differently? A shift toward the nonviolent language of partnership might begin with the nurse's ability to internally extend empathy to herself. You cannot give what you don't have. If you don't have empathy for yourself, then you cannot give it to others. A moment for self-empathy would have helped her connect in a more compassionate way with her patients. If the nurse understood how to use the tools of NVC she could have asked for a few minutes of empathy or she could have expressed herself in a way that may not have stimulated such a defensive reaction. This may have sounded like, "When I have heard five requests from you in the last thirty minutes, I feel stressed because I need some space to get my charting done. Would you be willing to go to your room and take care of your own needs for the next twenty minutes without asking me to help you?"

Domination-type language patterns block health care workers from offering the essential care the evolving system demands and hinder these workers from gaining the fulfillment that occurs when basic needs are met. At the organizational level, these language patterns prevent the development of the effective work forces needed to bring compassionate care to patients. By contrast, language that expresses the inner world of individuals—their feelings and needs—is less developed and may sound awkward as people struggle to verbalize their evolving awareness. As the system changes to one of partnership, however, language needs to change accordingly.

Partnerships Focused on Meeting Needs

Bringing NVC into organizations helps create language that supports the new worldview of partnership. This paradigm shift—from extrinsic to intrinsic motivation—leads to more accountability and staff who are more enthusiastic about what they do. At the same time, it fosters increased overall productivity and profitability. Problems such as fear of authority, resentful compliance, complacent entitlement, and cynicism—common within a domination system—are more readily resolved when the partnership model is embraced.

Using the tools of NVC gives organizations the ability to create and nurture more supportive, healing environments for both patients and staff. Language that expresses honesty and empathy, respect and understanding, appreciation and gratitude, mutuality and inclusion, supports "power with" structures that occur in partnership organizations.

A partnership system where the focus is on feelings and needs instead of titles creates a more egalitarian environment. In a partnership system, all needs are equal and everyone's feelings matter. If someone says or does something upsetting to you, it's OK to speak up and express your feelings. Speaking directly to the person who stimulated your reaction creates connections and prevents gossip and revenge.

I recall when I worked for a hospital where employees were taught to address their complaints directly to the offending person. This was scary at first but gradually got easier. The teams at this hospital were more effective than anyplace else I've worked, and this system helped me learn about the effects of my words on others. Remember the resident who was distressed over being thought "incompetent" because she was new and trying to learn? Imagine how the story might play out differently if she had expressed her feelings of distress directly to the Attending who judged her. The dynamic of judging the new person could begin to change and be replaced by a dynamic of understanding. Judgments are the opposite of understanding. Once people see your humanness and understand who you are, judgments dissolve.

What Does "Nonviolent" Mean?

People who have never heard of NVC may have a preconception about what constitutes violence. Most people think of violence in terms of physical aggression. In fact, physical violence often evolves from verbal violence. As you have seen in the discussion of the language of domination, verbal violence is often so unconscious and so culturally normal that people are not aware of the impact of the spoken word. You've begun to see that the words you use can create connection or disconnection. If I want to calm a patient down, I use words that focus on the person's feelings and needs. If someone is already upset and I use language that implies wrongness or makes a demand or threatens, I can expect that person to escalate and become physically violent.

When you talk about "Nonviolent" Communication then, you refer to deliberately using words that create connection and empowerment. Language that expresses blame, criticism, and judgment will often stimulate violence. Consider what happens inside of you when someone calls you a name. Do you feel angry or hurt because you are not being seen accurately? To be the recipient of this blaming, negative language without knowing how to get your own need for empathy met creates depression or anger. People are often surprised when a student takes a gun to school and shoots whoever is in range. Perhaps if this student had known how to verbalize his distress and had received empathy, he may not have tried to get his needs met in such a violent way.

Only through new language choices that reflect new beliefs and worldviews can you begin to resolve the wounds of the legacy of domination and pave the way to partnerships that work and heal.

Domination and Partnership, a Brief Review

In this chapter, you've looked at a number of differences between systems of domination and systems of partnership. As you read through the summary table below, think about where you are and where your workplace is in the process of evolution from Domination to Partnership. If you are like most of us, you can find many examples in your own experience of how relationships of dominance are very much at work in your life. Yet, perhaps you can also find examples of ways in which you, and the systems you are part of, have already begun to move toward the partnership model. In what areas do you feel the pull in that direction?

Until you become conscious of your own feelings and needs, and find your inner source of power, you are all pawns in the "domination system." If you continue to act unconsciously, you perpetuate the agenda of that system. As society evolves and people awaken to their true nature, the old tools of guilt, shame, and threats are no longer effective in motivating people. To use these tools with health care professionals insults their intelligence and creates hostility and resentment. "Intellectual capital will go where it is wanted, and it will stay where it is well treated. It cannot be driven; it can only be attracted."[4]

DOMINATION	PARTNERSHIP
Power over	Power with
Hierarchy of control	Moving toward conscientiousness
Obey, follow external orders	Authenticity, follow inner truth
Dominant and subordinate roles	We are each a complete whole
Based on fear	Based on trust
Creates dependency on external authorities	Creates empowerment and self-trust
Dependent, independent	Interdependent
Focus on extrinsic needs	Focus on intrinsic needs
Communicate to control others	Communicate to connect with others
Learning is a sign of weakness and lesser status	Learning is a responsibility and an ongoing need
Judge complex needs and wants and seek to force them into either/or categories: good/bad, right/wrong, strong/weak, appropriate/inappropriate	Accept the complexity of wants and needs and seek to understand them
Individuals serve the systems	Systems serve the individuals
Maintains status, caste system	Encourages respect and cooperation of all
Devalues needs for caring and empathy	Caring and empathy are highly valued
Dishonesty about needs sustains the system of authority	Honesty about needs sustains the partnership
Others held responsible for your actions and feelings	Personal responsibility for actions and feelings
Achieve status, then defend it	Ongoing evolution and growth
Life-alienating	Life-serving, life-enhancing
One right way	Respect for diverse beliefs
Life is cheap; categorize life	Life is sacred; revere all life

In the next chapter, you'll see some common language dynamics that occur in employee cultures within systems of domination, specifically nursing cultures. You'll also see how the same languages that diminish the quality of work environments for nurses also diminish the experience of care received by patients.

Notes: _____

1. Riane Eisler, *Sacred Pleasure* (New York: HarperCollins Publishers, 1995), p. 21.
2. Riane Eisler, *The Real Wealth of Nations*, Berrett-Koehler Publishers, Inc. 2007, pp. 30–31
3. Riane Eisler, *The Real Wealth of Nations*, p. 44.
4. Walter Wriston, former president and chairman of Citicorp. Author of *In the Twilight of Sovereignty: How the Information Revolution Is Transforming Our World* (New York: Charles Scribner's Sons, 1992).

Chapter 4

The Languages of Diagnosis, Judgment, Analysis, and Labeling

As you saw in Chapter 3, all organizations created in the image of the domination model rely on language patterns that emphasize hierarchy, and focus on controlling the world outside of yourself. Because Western medicine uses diagnosis and labeling as a basis for treatment, the languages of diagnosis, analysis, judgment, and labeling are particularly virulent in hospital cultures. Interestingly, these languages are not only directed at the patients they are used to "manage," they also come to permeate the interpersonal relationships between the people who work to provide care. In this chapter, you'll see more deeply what is meant by judgment, diagnosis, and labeling, consider the effects of these language patterns, and examine what it is about hospital systems that reinforces these processes. You'll also see what happens when you view these language processes through the lens of Nonviolent Communication (NVC), and explore the ways NVC can be used to improve the common negative dynamics of health care organizations.

The Principle of the Self-fulfilling Prophecy: How Judgments Trap and Limit You

When people judge and label you, a funny dynamic occurs. You begin to act out the judgments. When someone judges me as incompetent, I literally *become* incompetent. The tension and unease I feel around that person can prevent me from starting an IV or performing other tasks that I've done successfully in the past. I may drop things on the floor or say misleading things. When someone diagnoses me as unhelpful, the last thing I want to do is help that person. By contrast, when I am judged as competent, I feel more confident and it affects how I act. Labels, judgments, and diagnoses often become self-fulfilling prophecies.

Once you become what others have labeled you, the range of possibilities for your life narrows dramatically. In 1968, a schoolteacher named Jane Elliott did a remarkable study with her third grade class to show the effects of discrimination. She divided her class into two parts. One half was the "blue eyes" and the other, "brown eyes." One day, the blue eyes were treated in a judgmental and humiliating way, and the next day, the brown eyes were treated this way. The children in the low-status group performed poorly in the classroom. When they became the superior group, they performed well.

Three decades later, Oprah Winfrey repeated this experiment with her studio audience to similar effect. Even when the audience knew that they were part of an experiment, the group that was made to sit in a crowded room and wait at the back of the line felt hurt and angry, and conflict between the groups occurred. One member of the audience said that as soon as someone in power told him to treat the other group in a disrespectful way, he did it without thinking or challenging anyone. He went on to verbalize his understanding that it's the same thing that happened in Nazi Germany fifty years ago. Jane Elliott tells people that they have the power to change discrimination by changing their behavior, changing the words they say, and changing the way they think.

In this chapter, you'll examine how the phenomenon of the self-fulfilling prophecy—along with other phenomena associated with labeling, diagnosis, and judgment—impact everyone in health care systems: the people who work there, the patients they serve, and the organization as a whole.

How Diagnoses and Judgments Limit Organizational Effectiveness

When hospitals don't have harmonious work forces, everyone suffers. Workers suffer because a hostile environment creates stress and reduces motivation. Typically, sick leave increases and this creates stress on the administration as retention/recruitment costs skyrocket. And, in health care organizations, disharmony diminishes the quality of patient care as well, undermining the central service mission of the organization.

Judgments Undermine Staff Performance

When you work within environments that support judgment and labeling, you suffer from erosion of the quality of your performance. Your judgments of others actually diminish their ability to be effective in their work. The image below describes how judgment can trigger a chain reaction that culminates in behaviors that do not reflect your true potential competence.

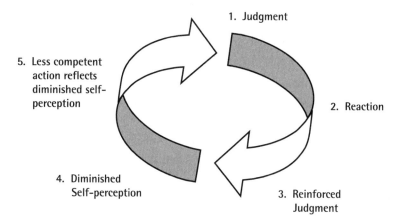

Let's walk through this cycle to see how it plays out in a health care setting. Let's say you are a new nurse on a unit and your colleague judges you to be incompetent, based on her assessment of your work history.

(Step 1) You react to her perception of your incompetence by dropping a sterile dressing on the floor.

(Step 2) The act of dropping the dressing reinforces her initial judgment.

(Step 3) You feel embarrassed and scared and your own perception of your competence is declining.

(Step 4) As an expression of your diminished confidence and increasing fearfulness, your hands shake while you change the dressing.

(Step 5) Now, the cycle repeats itself. The person observing you mentally labels you a "basket case."

(Step 1) You sense the judgment and begin to stutter when you are around that person.

(Step 2) This reinforces their judgment

(Step 3) which further undermines your confidence and self-esteem

(Step 4) causing you to second-guess every decision you make, which prevents you from finishing your work on time....

(Step 5) And around and around you go. You can see that the new nurse is on track to make a terrible mistake and perhaps even lose her job.

Cultures of Judgment Prevent Learning and Lead to Costly Errors

One of the first lessons I learned in nursing school was that "you are not allowed to make mistakes." Such an expectation creates an inhumane environment because you are all human, and humans make mistakes. When you try to be perfect, you become very rigid and treat yourself harshly.

This less than compassionate attitude toward yourself is reflected outward toward your colleagues. Instead of supporting someone when they make a mistake, they are judged. This creates hurt on top of fear and shame. It further increases the hostility of the workplace. Working in an environment that uses outwardly focused judgmental language and operates under a reward and punishment system does not meet employees' needs for compassion and safety. Workers are defensive and scared. Because communication is closed, emotional wounds cannot heal and a supportive community cannot be created.

Choosing Blame Over Learning

When nurses make a mistake, they often try to hide it because they fear punishment. For example, a nurse we'll call Lori made two medication errors and was called into the Head Nurse's office. The Head Nurse, understandably concerned about the safety of patients, told Lori that she could no longer distribute medications.

Instead of seizing an opportunity to learn about possible ways to improve the medication dispensing systems, the Head Nurse chose the "quick fix" route of blaming the nurse. As a result, Lori felt humiliated and her morale declined. When such things happen to one nurse, there is a trickle-down effect on everyone. The constant fear of making mistakes creates internal stress, which in turn increases the likelihood that mistakes will happen. Indeed, this is what happened to Lori. After she made the first medication error, she was so upset and frightened that she then made the second error.

Blaming people when they make a mistake prevents a deeper understanding of the issues and makes it more difficult to identify which systems are problems. When the nurse made the medication errors, placing blame on her prevented an examination of the medication system. If the focus had been on the system and the mistakes were recognized as a system breakdown, future mistakes could have been prevented.

What the Head Nurse Chose Not to Know

In fact, many factors contributed to the medication errors. For one thing, the medication book was a loose-leaf notebook and many of the pages had worked themselves loose from the rings and were falling out. Some of the handwriting was hard to read and there were so many discontinued medications mixed in with current medications that it was easy to miss a current medication that was due.

Not only that, on the day Lori made the second error, she'd been assigned two difficult patients and was responsible for giving out all the medications on the unit—and when the unit becomes busy, it is literally impossible to get everything done in the allotted time. On busy nights, the nurse who is distributing medications barely has time to talk to his or her assigned patients. If the assigned patients cannot care for themselves, it becomes highly likely that their care will be compromised or the medication they receive inaccurate.

When Lori complained to the administrator about the current medication system, the administrator said, "It works fine. It's the way we've always done it." Attachment to one strategy to accomplish a task will often result in problems especially if that strategy doesn't address human needs. What may seem like a good strategy for getting a task done actually isn't, if it causes worker stress.

Why Would Lori Choose Not to Self-report?

Another problem with medication systems such as the one I'm describing has to do with retaliation. A nurse who discovers a medication error (or any kind of error) is supposed to report it to the supervisor and write an incident report. If she does this and the person making the error gets in trouble, then some kind of retaliation occurs. The person who got in trouble watches the "informant" looking for any excuse to get her in trouble. This adds to the hostile environment and prevents cooperation and friendship between staff members. Nurses need to watch their backs as well as their fronts.

Resentment occurs when you do something for someone because you are afraid of the consequences. By contrast, when you take action and give because you have compassion for others' needs, you create an environment of trust and harmony. An essential ingredient for team building is recognizing others' needs and realizing that everyone has a unique gift to contribute. However, the language of judgment blocks communication so that recognizing others' needs and contributions cannot occur.

How Communication Habits Create Negative Nursing Cultures

Why Are Working Relationships Among Nurses So Often Troubled?

In Lori's story, you began to explore a number of the dynamics that lead to troubled working relationships between nurses. In Lori's interactions with her Head Nurse around her medication errors, you saw a microcosm of the ways in which performance is undermined by habits of blame and judgment in moments where compassion-based learning would serve the organization better.

Let's look more deeply now at the world of nursing as an example of how the systems you live in reflect and perpetuate your beliefs about one another and your sense of what is possible. Whether or not the labels fit, nurses are widely thought to be unsupportive toward one another, often judgmental, and even backstabbing. Because of their habitual communication style, they often alienate one another, creating disharmony and separation. Nurses want to work together harmoniously, but when you look carefully at the structures under which nurses work, it becomes understandable why they sometimes create negative work cultures.

Nurses experience extraordinary levels of stress in their working environments. Working with sick people is emotionally taxing work. Patients in the hospital are in crisis, which places stress on their family or social systems. Patients often express their distress in ways that can be interpreted as hostile, and their families also express their distress toward the health care team in ways that can be difficult to deal with compassionately. The system of identifying a particular person in a family system as the mentally ill one can create uncomfortable dynamics for the nursing staff. When a person is labeled as mentally ill, it lets the family off the hook. Families don't need to look inside themselves to their own pathology or understand the family dynamics that contributed to their ill family member's problem because they believe that the identified patient has a chemical imbalance, which is the cause of his or her problem. When nurses interact with the patient and the family do not like or understand what they are doing, the family will often judge the nurse as doing something wrong and will fire the nurse from taking care of their family member. At no point does the family have the motivation to begin to look at how they think and communicate because the labeling system that is in place in medicine reinforces their own system of judging and thinking in terms of right and wrong. This prevents them from doing the healing work on themselves that is essential if the patient has any hope of getting well.

Organizational issues also frequently create stresses. Frequent staffing shortages and the communications dynamics discussed here make it especially difficult to maintain a positive attitude. Many nurses stay on in the health care system even after they have become burnt out. They are emotionally exhausted from their struggles of being a caregiver, in a system where they are not respected. They have played out the role of the "good" nurse who gives up her/his needs to care for the needs of others, and they have lost themselves in the process.

These multiple stressors can easily create troubled interpersonal dynamics. When people are stressed, they tend to lash out at one another. In an attempt to locate pain outside of themselves, workers find someone with less status to judge and criticize. Instead of taking responsibility for their feelings and communicating their needs directly (habits that are not cultivated in domination systems, as you've seen), people create a scapegoat.

Diagnosing and Labeling Your Co-workers: A Recipe for Disharmony

Nurses and other staff members label and diagnose patients and this habit spills into their interpersonal relationships with colleagues; they also label and diagnose one another. Patterns of labeling and diagnosis are applied to everyone on the team and the culture abounds with efforts to categorize co-workers with overly simple labels like good and bad, right and wrong, normal and abnormal, competent and incompetent, sane and crazy.

When I started working on the psychiatric unit, for example, I felt nervous when I heard the language of labels, diagnoses, and judgments being used. The employees seemed attached to thinking in that way. They had the sanctity of the system behind them. I knew it was only a matter of time before I would be labeled and judged because when people think in terms of labels and judgments they generalize that thinking to include everyone.

Indirect Communication Reinforces Judgments

A system of indirect communication is widespread among health care workers. This dynamic contributes to what is most often called "back-stabbing." Instead of speaking directly to the person someone has a problem with, the employee gripes about that person to someone else. The individual they are griping to, lacking knowledge and tools about how to deal effectively with the situation, usually ends up colluding with the griping person (collusion occurs when there is agreement with another person's judgments). Now instead of one person holding judgment about another, two people are in judgment. Instead of clearing up the problem, the environment becomes filled with "bad vibes." Not surprisingly, people sense and are uncomfortable around someone in judgment of them.

Hierarchies Compound the Labeling Problem

Hierarchies in the nursing structure can be additional barriers to effective communication. The differences in status conferred by the hierarchy can too easily be used to justify the patterns of judgment and indirect communication that permeate nursing cultures. As you come to believe that the structural hierarchy reflects real differences in talent, skill, or worth (as opposed to being just an organizational tool), you become unable to recognize that the people at the bottom of the hierarchy may have just as much to contribute as those at the top.

For example, a Charge Nurse said to me the other evening: "We are not equal. I've worked here a lot longer than you, and I know a whole lot more than you do." This Charge Nurse has become enmeshed in the system and was using the status conferred by the organizational hierarchy to justify an attitude of unwillingness to learn. She does not empower the staff to do their job but creates dependence by making their decisions for them (because, after all, she knows more than they do). She also does not enable open communications because people don't feel safe expressing their truth to someone who uses his or her position to punish or put others down. If this Charge Nurse realized what her underlying need was (perhaps for acknowledgment and appreciation), then she'd be able to ask for that in a more direct way—thus acting as a positive role model and creating more open communication on the unit.

Labels Become Excuses for Poor Performance

Earlier, in the discussion of the dynamic of the self-fulfilling prophecy, I talked about how labeling others places limits on their performance. In systems where labels and diagnoses are rampant, they can also be used by individuals to justify their counterproductive behaviors. For instance, I was once at a meeting in which a fellow staff member said, "I have ADHD, so it's OK that I interrupt. I can't help it." She had identified with the label ADHD and now used it as a reason to continue acting in ways that did not benefit herself or others. In accepting the label ADHD, this staff member made a choice to perpetuate behaviors that diminished her ability to be perceived as a constructive member of a working team. This kind of self-limiting and team-limiting labeling could only be tolerated in a system that accepts diagnostic labels as "facts" rather than stories you tell in efforts to manage and control complex experiences.

The negative impacts of labeling and judgment on working relationships among nurses are numerous. These dynamics also profoundly impact the emotional health of individual nurses and other caregivers in health care settings.

Judgment Turned Inward Creates Depression

Judging isn't something you simply project outward: to the same extent as you judge others, so do you judge yourself. Thus when someone calls me "a hopeless neurotic," I collude with them, becoming fixated on what is wrong with me. If I make a mistake, I label myself "idiot." When people turn this judgmental language inward, they often become depressed. When they turn the language outward, they can become violent.

Depression is a wake-up call to tell you that your needs are not being met. To heal, you must feel.

Feelings are like the warning signals on your car. They point to a problem, a belief system, a way of thinking, or an unmet need. You wouldn't cut the cable to the warning signal on your car so you could ignore the problem, but it is standard practice to label feelings as being the problem and numb them out with medication. Medications blunt your feelings, preventing you from accessing and healing the underlying problem.

In order to heal depression or other disorders, you need to change the underlying beliefs that create unwanted symptoms or behaviors. As I journeyed through my own depression, I changed my lifestyle and started paying attention to what would meet my needs. I identified my thoughts and beliefs that kept me stuck in a depressive state. It was tempting for me to buy into the idea that I had a chemical imbalance and that I could not help being depressed. It would have been a relief to think that my depression was outside of my control. I could have taken the medication that the doctor gave me and limited my life based on a false belief that I was sick.

Instead, I learned the process of NVC that helped me adjust my belief systems to a more compassionate paradigm. I did inner work that included expressing deep feelings in a group setting where others received me with empathy. This allowed me to release pent-up emotions and helped me to embrace my own feelings and experiences without judging them. In order to express my pain to others, I had to overcome a deeply ingrained family rule: "Don't air your dirty laundry in public." Dirty laundry was any truth that had to do with unmet needs. It is impossible to get empathy for unmet needs if you are not allowed to talk about them. If you do not bring the pain that gets stimulated when needs are not met out into the light, then that pain festers inside and is expressed in less conscious ways (such as physical illness, homicidal rage, and self destruction.) Expressing my pain to others in a vulnerable way was difficult because I was stuck in thinking in terms of right and wrong. It had been drilled into me that airing my dirty laundry was wrong so when I did it, I felt ashamed. If I hadn't been in touch with the healing and relief that occurred when I got empathy, I would not have persisted in my efforts.

This illustrates that many of your cultural beliefs prevent you from doing the very things you need to do in order to heal. I contend that the language you speak (that of judgments, blame, and labels) creates outward violence toward others or inward violence toward yourself. It is not a surprise that antidepressants are one of the bestselling medications on the market.

The Myth of "Selfish Needs"

Some nurses believe that to admit they have needs is to be selfish. When I spoke at a hospice conference one year, a participant was very upset when I suggested that nurses should put their own needs first. She could not understand how nurses could put their needs before the needs of a dying person.

It may seem paradoxical that patients will actually receive more compassionate care if the nurse puts her own needs first. If the nurse does not take care of her needs, then she will begin to feel resentful, angry, and depressed. If a nurse cares for her own needs first, she will have more energy to care for others.

The average time that a nurse works for a hospice is one year. I believe the high burnout rate is directly related to the myth that you should give up your needs and take care of the needs of others. Many nurses who have become burnt out feel sad because they enjoy contributing to others and would like to be able to continue serving people with a positive attitude. They would do well to realize that by caring for their own needs first, they'd be freer to express their natural compassion and may better enjoy caring for others.

You've looked at how the communication patterns of judgment, diagnosis, and labeling diminish organizational effectiveness, create negative working relationships between nurses, and undermine the emotional well-being of individual caregivers. All of these negative effects, of course, contribute to the biggest concern of all: how these communication patterns actually undermine patient health, and work against the organizational mission of healing.

How Diagnoses And Labels Prevent Patient Healing

The Problem With Diagnosis

Diagnosis can be useful in treating disease. However, attachment to thinking in terms of what someone *is* can prevent health care providers from creating effective treatments that address not only the disease but the whole person. A diagnosis is really just an educated guess. It labels a group of symptoms. It does not deal with the cause of the symptoms nor does it tease apart the psychological, physiological, and emotional factors that contribute to the problem.

As you learn more and more about the complex connections between your minds, bodies, and spirits, the limitations of traditional diagnosis become clearer. Even the Center for Disease Control (CDC) agrees that there is an emotional component to 85 percent of diseases. Other doctors and scientists who have expanded beyond conventional approaches to medicine claim that a person's current health status is 100 percent connected to his or her mental and emotional reactions to the events of life. Treating the symptoms of a disease and ignoring the underlying emotional cause perpetuates a limited, band-aid approach to medicine.

Focusing only on treating symptoms not only ignores the underlying causes of disease, the symptom-diagnosis model often weakens a person's ability to heal. A common example is the person who experiences anxiety and is diagnosed on a spectrum of anxiety disorders. To address the symptom of anxiety, she takes an anti-anxiety drug. As time progresses, she does not deal with the cause of her anxiety but continues to suppress it by using more and more drugs. As she becomes addicted to drugs, she learns a way of coping that sets her up to be dependent on a "fix" outside of herself in order to survive. She loses or fails to find the inner empowerment that would allow her to find the source of her anxiety and heal it.

Labels Create Distance

The diagnosis habit impacts patients by reducing their full humanity to a set of symptoms. When caregivers are trained to think in terms of labels, judgments, diagnoses, and analyses, they become disconnected from their natural state of compassion and can dehumanize others. Labels and judgments create separations between caregivers and their own nature, and between them and their patients. The act of labeling sets up an *us* vs. *them* mentality which makes it possible to treat *them* in ways that *we* would not want to be treated ourselves.

For example, patients are routinely referred to by their diagnosis, i.e., "the schizophrenic in room 33" or "the diabetic in room 552." Such distancing, dehumanizing language reduces complex human beings into cases and problems and in the process disconnects you from your own feelings and needs.

The dehumanization process that relies on labels to manage and control others is more than just distancing, it does a kind of violence to its targets. Communicating in terms of labels, judgments, diagnoses, and analyses is violent (even if passively so) because it triggers pain and fear in others. Such passive violence is more insidious than physical violence because it generates anger in people who instinctively recoil at being dehumanized in this way. That anger, when turned outward, culminates in physical violence and turned inward culminates in depression. The way you communicate can become fuel for anger and violence—or it can create peace and harmony.

What Happens When Someone Buys Into the Labels and Diagnosis Placed on Them by the Medical System?

Unfortunately, most people are extremely vulnerable to the diagnoses of doctors. Domination systems socialize people to obey and agree with authority figures. When someone in a position of power, such as a doctor, says something, people believe him or her.

The following examples demonstrate the many ways this habitual use of labeling language damages patients. Sue is a disabled woman who has been in the psychiatric unit several times since I have worked there. She is usually admitted after suicide attempts. One day, she spent the morning screaming. A nurse asked her what she was screaming about and she said, "I'm crazy, so it's OK to act like this." Upon hearing this, the nurse said to her colleagues, "She shows good insight." "Good insight" in this unit means that the patient agrees with the unit's diagnosis and labels.

On another occasion, when Sue was headed to bed, the nurse reminded her to use the toilet before lying down. Sue said, "I'm lazy, so I'm going to wet the bed." She refused to use the bathroom, and wet the bed. Sue had been called "lazy" by people and so became that label.

In a conversation about her future, another patient informed me that she had decided not to pursue a relationship with her significant other because of her bipolar disorder. I asked her what she planned on doing when she was discharged from the hospital. She said she would clean her parents' house and do the laundry. I was sad to think that her identification with the label "bipolar" had so dramatically begun to narrow her sense of possibilities and life choices. Looking into this woman's future, it was not hard to imagine how the self-imposed limitations of remaining in service to her parents could ultimately make her less well rather than healthier.

I reflected on my own experience with depression. When I was depressed, the more I stopped myself from doing something because of my depression, the more depressed I became. As I focused on what was wrong with me I became more of that, but when I started focusing on my dreams and on what I wanted, I moved in that direction.

Because labels create such a compelling reality, they also prevent you from seeing the truth and hobble your capacity to perceive creative and healing possibilities. In her book *Kitchen Table Wisdom*, Dr. Naomi Remen puts it this way:

> Labeling sets up an expectation of life that is often so compelling that we can no longer see things as they really are. This expectation often gives us a false sense of familiarity toward something that is really new and unprecedented. Actually we are in relationship with our expectations, not with life itself. This suggests that we may become as wounded by the way in which we see an illness as by the illness itself. Belief traps or frees us….[1]

Naomi Ramen says that she bought into her doctor's label of Crohn's Disease and his assumptions that because of her illness, she could not possibly lead a productive life. As a result, she doubted herself and began canceling speaking engagements and decreasing her workload. "The power of the expert is very great and the way in which an expert sees you may easily become the way in which you see yourself."[2]

The Language of Diagnosis Denies the Reality of Life's Fluidity

The language of analyses, judgments, diagnoses, and labels is a "static language." It is destructive and creates conflict because life is not static. Life is a process. Naomi Remen, M.D., conveys this beautifully:

> Naming a disease has limited usefulness. It does not capture life or even reflect it accurately. Illness, on the

other hand, is a process, like life is. Much in the
concept of diagnosis and cure is about fixing, and a
narrow-bore focus on fixing people's problems can lead
to denial of the power of their process.[3]

To communicate in an accurate, healing way, you need a "process
language," such as NVC, which recognizes that people are growing and
changing all the time.

In psychiatry, diagnoses and labels are expressed in a way that
makes them final. When I was diagnosed as depressed, the psychiatrist
said, "You'll have to take medication the rest of your life." When a
person in a position of authority makes such a definitive statement, you
should be concerned. Many factors contribute to depression, yet the
psychiatrist was looking only at the symptoms and the accepted medical
treatment. Granted, the psychiatrist was trying to help me. He was
acting under the belief system that depression is a physical illness that
can lead to death by suicide. The information he was basing his actions
on was the most up-to-date research available.

I appreciate his effort but I cannot help remembering that
treatments such as mercury were used in the past to treat certain
disorders. Mercury was the accepted treatment at that time. Now you
know that mercury is toxic, and you would not think of prescribing it.
Because knowledge and scientific research is always evolving, I would
rather trust the wisdom that is present in my being. I prefer to believe
that your bodies and your minds have the ability to heal themselves.
With proper emotional support, nurturing, and nutrition, most diseases
can reverse themselves. Healing yourself is more about a shift in
consciousness and inspired action rather than finding the right pill.

People's feelings can change from second to second. To even begin
to communicate the fluidity of those feelings, you need to change the
way you've been taught to think and communicate. Naomi Remen
makes the distinction between using a static approach to medicine and
a process one. She says, "Seeing the life force in human beings brings
medicine closer to gardening than to carpentry. I don't fix a rosebush. A
rosebush is a living process, and as a student of that process I can learn

to prune, to nurture and cooperate with it in ways that allow it best to 'happen,' to maximize the life force in it even in the presence of disease."[4]

The direct negative effects on patients caused by diagnosis and static language are compounded by the indirect impacts of the nursing cultures you explored earlier in this chapter.

Nurses' Habitual Communication Patterns Negatively Impact Patient Care

The truth is that patients suffer when nurses don't work well together to harmonize their care. Patients are adversely affected when a stressed-out employee acts in an impatient, curt, or even offensive way toward them. Their lives can even be endangered when communication dynamics within the system create unhealthy reactions.

For example, one year Marshall Rosenberg was invited to work with a group of hospital nurses who had been forgetting to do a very important procedure in the Operating Room. The Head Nurse had told the nurses repeatedly to do this procedure, emphasizing that they had no choice but to do it. When Dr. Rosenberg talked to the nurses about why they didn't follow the procedure, they initially said, "We forget." When probed deeper, the nurses admitted that they felt considerable resentment toward the Head Nurse and were angry at the dictatorial way she expressed her requests. When the nurses heard her demands, they experienced a conflict between head and heart, which made them "forget" to do what she asked. Once the Head Nurse learned how to make requests that respected the emotional life of the nurses, the dynamic of "forgetting" was resolved.

Nurses Lack the Communication Tools to Meet Patients' Emotional Needs

Most nurses want to help others, yet the communication tools they use often prevent them from meeting the emotional needs of the patient.

Instead of understanding what motivates a person to act in a certain way and instead of using language that captures the patient's present feelings and needs, nurses use habitual communication patterns such as advice-giving. This puts them in a precarious position. If the patient acts on this advice and has a bad outcome, then the nurse will be blamed.

Giving advice also disrespects a patient's ability to find their own answers. It perpetuates their sense of helplessness and can often stimulate defensive reactions. Advice blocks communication; it often attempts to solve the problem before getting to the root of it. Health care workers, by assuming that patients need fixing, don't take the time to check out what the underlying need is. Your very assumptions block communications and prevent you from seeing the true picture.

Checking out patients' underlying needs could save money and lives. The process would begin from the understanding that patients themselves are not always clear about what their needs are and why they are seeking help. Many years ago, I went to see my doctor because I was having heart arrhythmias. I was distressed because I had just ended a relationship. I knew my arrhythmias were a manifestation of my distress, and realized as I left the doctor's office that what I really needed was empathy for my emotional pain. My doctor knew I was distressed when I expressed my emotional pain to her, but instead of empathizing with me, she gave me a prescription for a heart medication. She was focusing on the diagnosis of heart arrhythmias and the standard treatment for that instead of focusing on my underlying human need. I never filled the prescription and, with the support of friends who were able to give me empathy, my arrhythmias went away. Until the underlying need is heard clearly, your best intentions to help others can cause more harm than good.

Returning to the Source: Feelings and Needs

You've seen how judgment creates distance between human beings and enables you to act in ways that dehumanize others. You've also looked at how judgments, when codified as labels, can trap you in false realities, undermine your competence, prevent learning, and limit the range of possibilities you can see for your futures and yourself.

Given the negative consequences of judgment and labeling, you might wonder what it is that keeps you so tied to this pattern of communication. Why do you continue to express yourself in ways that do such harm? The answer has everything to do with your learned difficulty in taking responsibility for and directly expressing your authentic feelings and needs—those core personal truths that are so suppressed within domination systems.

Why Do You Perpetuate This Judging Habit?

None of you can heal your own perceptions of reality until you realize that other people don't cause your feelings. Only by taking responsibility for your feelings can you quit judging and blaming and begin communicating in a life-serving way. Others can *trigger* your feelings, but the origin of feelings lies within your needs. When you hold onto judgments, instead of owning your own feelings and asking for what you want, you create enemy images of others and create disharmony and confusion.

Dr. Marshal Rosenberg says that all labels, analyses, and judgments of others are tragic expressions of your own unmet needs.[5] They are tragic expressions because when people express needs in this indirect way, it creates defensive reactions in others that virtually assure that the needs will not be met.

Can you imagine wanting to help a supervisor who says to her staff: "You are too selfish to care about anyone but yourself?" When a supervisor uses this kind of language, those around her are likely to react out of fear, shame, guilt, or obligation. Goodwill toward her decreases and resentment increases. But what is this supervisor really saying? What is the unmet need she is expressing by making this accusation of others? Is she really saying, "I'm hurting here and need assistance" or "I'm afraid that my needs for support and understanding will not be met"?

Many of you do not realize that when you judge or label others you are revealing information about yourself, not about the person you are judging. When this supervisor calls her staff "selfish," she is not describing a truth about them (though, as you've seen, it might *become* the truth through the dynamics of the self-fulfilling prophecy). Everyone has his or her own interpretation of others. What one person judges as "selfish" another could judge as "self-directed." The real truth she is expressing by labeling her colleagues "selfish" is her own distress, which was triggered by something that one or more of her colleagues did.

The cycle of labeling and reaction leads the supervisor and her staff down a rabbit trail of false reality. As they all focus their energy on reacting to the label "selfish," they are getting further and further from the core issue—the supervisor's feelings and needs.

Your tendency to focus your attention outward also distracts you from taking responsibility for your own feelings and needs. Let's say I'm explaining a procedure to my co-worker, George. I can tell that George doesn't understand what I'm saying, and I begin to form a judgment that crystallizes in the label "George is stupid." The next day, my co-worker, Amy, is trying to explain a new computer system to me, and I'm just not getting it. Flipping into my habit of judgment, I tell myself "Amy is a lousy communicator." By projecting my judgments outward, I've created for myself the experience of being surrounded by stupid people who cannot communicate.

But, what if I assumed responsibility for my own feelings and needs? What if, in my interaction with George, I was able to partner with him by saying, "I'm feeling frustrated that I'm not communicating this in a way that you can understand—what do you think might help?" What if, in my interaction with Amy, I was able to say, "Amy, I'm feeling overwhelmed by all this new information at once, and a little scared that I'm not going to master it all today. Would you be willing to slow down a little, and maybe plan some time tomorrow to review after I've had a chance to come up with some questions?" Suddenly, instead of feeling surrounded by stupid people who cannot communicate, I'm partnering with others to get my own needs met.

Changing the outward focus of labels and judgments to an inward orientation of feelings and needs could revolutionize the health care system. When health care workers take responsibility for their own feelings instead of projecting them on others in the form of judgments, labels, and analyses, hospital environments will become more supportive places to work, and staff effectiveness will expand.

Compassion Begins at Home

A key insight of NVC is that the more compassionate you are with yourself, the more compassion you have for others. When you judge and criticize yourself, you are likely to judge and criticize others. What is within is also without.

A graduate nurse undergoing orientation on a psychiatric unit expressed her distress to me about the way she was treated and the way she was expected to treat patients. She explained that using power over tactics and control measures is not in harmony with her internal values. She asked, "How does one remain human working in this environment?"

How *does* a nurse remain human working in an environment that is not supportive of both patients and staff? How *does* one maintain an open heart in the midst of systems that communicate via judgments and labels? When you find yourself struggling within such a system, the natural reaction is to shut down and protect yourself. When you do this, you lose touch with your compassion and spend your energy protecting yourself instead of helping others.

There is another way. You can learn new communication tools so you can see the heart of others and help build the heart of the institution to better serve its staff and patients. By realizing that people express feelings and needs in judgmental ways, you can become skilled at not taking things personally. If nurses could learn not to take things personally and if they received support from management, and from one another, their jobs would be easier. If they could offer empathy to one another and to patients, then hospitals could become healing environments for patients and for employees. Only by expressing your honesty and your discomfort about how systems of domination affect you, will you contribute to the evolution of the institutions in which you work.

Notes: _____

1. Naomi Remen, M.D., *Kitchen Table Wisdom* (New York: Berkley Publishing Group, 1996), p. 66.
2. Naomi Remen, M.D., *Kitchen Table Wisdom*, p. 235.
3. Naomi Remen, M.D., *Kitchen Table Wisdom*, pp. 223–24.
4. Naomi Remen M.D., *Kitchen Table Wisdom*, p. 225.
5. Marshall Rosenberg, Ph.D., *Nonviolent Communication, A Language of Life*, second edition (Encinitas, California: PuddleDancer Press, 2003), p. 16.

Chapter 5

From "Power Over" to "Power With": The Case of Psychiatric Medicine

As you seek to understand and recognize the negative impacts of domination practices on your health care organizations, your lives as health care providers, and your patients' health, the world of psychiatric medicine offers a fascinating case study. The dynamics of domination are heightened in the psychiatric unit environment, in part because psychiatric medicine aims to treat not only the bodies, but also the behaviors of the patients. In this chapter, you'll look at the ways that traditional psychiatry models perpetuate violence and create unsafe environments for those who are ill and those who would help them recover. In a time when hospitals are increasingly recognizing the limitations of control and punishment tactics, you'll also explore what the Nonviolent Communication (NVC) model can teach you about how to create safer, more humane environments for the treatment of psychiatric illnesses.

Control and Punishment Tactics Create Danger, Not Safety

For generations, the models of psychiatric medicine have relied heavily on tools of control, domination, reward, and punishment. The assumption has been that safer environments are created when psychiatric patients are kept "under control" through systems of restraint, reward and punishment, including violent punishment. In this classic model, psychiatric patients are viewed as rebellious children who, in order to become better, must submit to the control of medical expert adults who have diagnosed what is wrong and can fix it only if the "child" complies.

The domination-based adult/child relationship is compounded by the entrenched power of labeling that so permeates psychiatric medicine. In no area of medicine is the practice of diagnosis and labeling (discussed at length in Chapter 4) more powerfully at work. Indeed, the core competency of psychiatric staff lies in correctly labeling Axis I or Axis II characteristics. Preconceived notions about patients based on these labeling systems drive the philosophy and systems embedded in traditional psychiatric units everywhere, and they define and limit the range of possibilities for a patient's care.

The problem is that the tactics of control and the practices of labeling simply don't work well. Statistics show that psychiatric staffs are assaulted more often than police officers, and staff and patients alike have expressed concerns about inhumane treatment of patients. Indeed, hospitals are under pressure from JACHO, the accrediting board for hospitals, to avoid control and punishment tactics. In particular, the use of restraints and seclusion to control patients are increasingly under scrutiny. Unfortunately, hospitals tend to be reactive instead of proactive. It often takes a crisis, such as a patient who dies in restraints, before leaders are willing to entertain innovative strategies that will change the way they operate.

Teaching NVC can help hospitals obtain and sustain accreditation by integrating verbal de-escalation techniques and encouraging staff to create compassionate relationships with patients. By encouraging cooperation instead of hostility and violence, shifting the way you think about others from a labeling system to an empathic system, and employing different tools, it is possible to create more humane environments that are safer and better aligned with the evolving philosophy of health care institutions.

Changing Your Beliefs About Mental Illness

As you begin to more deeply understand the flaws in the domination model of psychiatric medicine and begin to embrace a nonviolent partnership model, it is increasingly easy to see how blind you've become to the range of possibilities for treating mental illness. Mental health institutions mirror the Western beliefs about mental health, including the belief that mental illness exists within an autonomous individual and is a consequence of an individual's personal physiology. But this is not the only way to think about mental illness.

In fact there are many strategies for treating mental illness. One culture successfully treats "mentally ill" children by removing them from their family of origin and placing them with another family. The children improve until they're placed back with their family of origin at which point they tend to regress. This raises a fundamental question: are most so-called "mental illnesses" really physiological conditions (as the pharmaceutical industry claims), or are they self-protective mechanisms you learn in order to cope with unnatural and unhealthy conditions? How this question is answered plays into your basic, underlying belief systems. Your answers, in turn, affect the strategies you choose for treating conditions such as depression, schizophrenia, attention-deficit disorder, and others, and how you organize mental health institutions.

If you believe mental illness is a physiological condition and think there's something wrong with the individual, you build health care systems like the ones you have now. If on the other hand you believe "mental illness" is a systems problem, you'll create health care systems that focus on healing rather than pathology.

Changing the structure of institutions will change the outcome. In the current system, you see patients who become "institutionalized." They are taught how to get their needs met in a system that stresses pathology and uses domination strategies to control them. Changing the underlying belief system that classifies mental illness as physiological will change the strategies used to treat it and will radically improve the outcomes of care.

"Protective" Versus "Punitive" Use of Force

Before going further with a discussion of violence and control in the context of psychiatric medicine, it is critical to acknowledge the differences between punitive use of force and protective use of force. At times, force may be necessary to prevent a patient from harming him- or herself or others. This is the protective use of force. Punitive force, by contrast, is when force is used as a punishment if the patient does not comply with a staff person's demand. Through their actions, staff who use punitive force reveal that they lack the tools to create the type of connection that leads to harmony and cooperation.

An example of the use of protective force occurred recently on the unit where I work. One evening, a twenty-three-year-old female patient made a weapon out of a plastic fork. She was using it to cut her arms and abdomen. There was blood all over the room and the patient fought anyone who tried to take the weapon away. It took six people to subdue her and put her in restraints.

When such a dramatic event occurs, it is useful to review the intentions of the patient from an NVC perspective. The NVC model begins with the understanding that people's actions and communication patterns are oriented to meeting their needs. Perhaps this patient was trying to meet needs for:

1. relief from emotional pain (cutting releases endorphins);
2. attention (she got a lot of attention);
3. power (she was in control at least for awhile); and
4. safety (by being in restraints, the patient felt safe).

By identifying and honoring the needs this patient was expressing through her self-damaging actions, you can begin to figure out alternative ways those needs might be met. As long as you condemn or ignore the needs underlying the behavior, you make no real intervention in the larger pattern of self-damaging actions. Further, I suspect this young woman's strategy of cutting herself would not have occurred if the unit had addressed her needs earlier and if the unit was set up to support "power with" relationships with patients instead of "power over" relationships.

A History of Power Over Tactics

The traditional model of psychiatry emphasizes drug therapy and a patient/doctor relationship in which the doctor or therapist is personally invisible. This is different from a humanistic or transpersonal approach to healing. The philosopher Martin Buber asserts that healing cannot occur between a patient and a therapist. It can only occur, he explained, between equal people whose hearts are open to each other. He calls this the "I-Thou relationship." The I-Thou relationship occurs when there is mutuality, openness, directness, and presence.[1]

Buber's vision of the therapeutic value of mutual and open relationships are a far cry from the way relationships are structured in a traditional psych unit. Patients in a traditional setting learn quickly that their "success" depends on their willingness to submit to the staff members whose job it is to dominate them. If they do not voluntarily do what a staff person tells them to do, they'll be forced to do it.

For instance, if a patient refuses to take his antipsychotic medications, he'll be held down by several staff members and injected with medication. If he refuses to go to his room when asked, security officers will be called to forcibly put him in his room. These power over tactics combined with strong medications effectively repress the patient so that he quits "acting out." Once he is sufficiently repressed, he's deemed in good behavioral control and sent to another unit or discharged.

And then what happens? It's no surprise that patients get in one crisis after another when they leave the hospital and often make repeat trips back to the unit. While in the hospital, patients don't learn new ways of being or new ways of meeting their deepest needs so they perpetuate their existing patterns of reacting to life's challenges and get into trouble over and over again. Medication and control tactics suppress selected behaviors; they don't address the underlying causes of those behaviors.

People Can Only Change When They Have the Choice

Where else but in psychiatry can a patient be locked into a hospital against his or her own will? This act of violence toward people prevents healing from occurring because it creates resistance. People need to have choice in order to grow and heal. You cannot force anyone to do anything. You can only punish them if they don't. Taking away a person's choice stimulates feelings of powerlessness and anger. Instead of empowering people, it creates dependency. Punishment also stimulates anger and sometimes retaliation. This creates an unsafe environment for staff and for patients.

For the system of involuntary commitment to change, the society needs to create healthy, healing alternatives where patients who are a danger to themselves or others can go and receive compassionate care. I envision small healing centers where distressed people can go and receive healthy food, compassionate care, and education in self-care and healing modalities. Hospitals can create a more nurturing environment by training their staff in NVC and building different types of healing modalities and education into their program. Patients at the hospital I work at are very interested in NVC when I talk with them about it. I suspect if it were a regular part of the program that patients would enjoy using the tools to grow and heal.

Removing Choice Creates Resistance

In my experiences working in psychiatric units, I've had many opportunities to notice how the more traditional approach affects others. The nurses I work with who are immersed in power over thinking often create dynamics that contribute to the violence of the unit. For example, one night the Charge Nurse had placed my assigned patient in seclusion while I was off the unit with another patient (seclusion is when a patient is locked in his or her room). When I came back, I wanted to go into the patient's room and talk to him. The Charge Nurse said, "Don't go in there, he'll rush the door."

The patient wanted to come out of his room, so as I spoke with him through the locked door, I asked him if he'd be willing to sit on the bed. He agreed to do this, demonstrating that he could cooperate with staff requests. I again spoke with the Charge Nurse and asked that I be allowed to go into the room and talk with the patient. The Charge Nurse still felt uncomfortable about opening the door. So I told the patient that I appreciated his cooperation but was unable to open his door right now because the Charge Nurse felt nervous about his ability to control his behavior.

The Charge Nurse snapped at me when she heard this, saying, "Don't tell him I'm nervous, tell him that when he's a good boy, you'll open the door." I perceived such a statement as an indication of the philosophy that the unit operates from. Instead of developing "power with" the patients, the staff creates distance through power over tactics. They don't realize that by hiding their own humanity from the patients, they create an "us vs. them" environment that inhibits cooperation and healing.

When you talk down to patients, you increase the likelihood of violence because all people need to be treated with respect. When you don't meet people's needs, their behavior escalates in an attempt to get these needs met. Patients often act in violent ways trying to get their needs met because they don't understand what their own needs are and have no tools for meeting these needs in healthier ways. When the staff responds "violently" to patients through verbal or physical "power over" tactics, the environment remains hostile. Cooperation and healing does not occur.

When the Maximum Security Unit at Mendota Medical Center integrated NVC into their program, not only did the use of restraints and seclusion decrease, but patients and staff also began to empathize with one another. During the tornado season, the hospital has drills where patients get locked in their rooms. Usually this stimulates violent behavior by the patients and a trying shift for the staff. This year, however, the patients were quiet and cooperative. When asked what had changed, the patients responded by saying, "The staff are not into power and control anymore. They don't like locking us in our room anymore than we like it."

Applying Empathy Tools to a Patient in Distress Will De-escalate Tension and Create "Power With" Them

The use of empathy will begin to establish a trusting connection so that nonviolent solutions to problems can occur instead of power struggles. By contrast, ignoring patients' needs for empathy and dignity creates resistance. An example of this dynamic occurred one night on my unit. A young woman I'll call Paula was brought in after threatening to commit suicide. Paula was extremely angry upon being placed in our locked unit. She said, "This place is like a jail. I feel like I'm being punished." There were three staff members nearby and the patient pointed to me and said, "I want to speak with you." (She had been on our unit before and my guess is that she pointed at me this time because she sensed I'd deal with her in a compassionate way.)

I began to empathize with Paula's point of view and she calmed down slightly. I could feel a nice connection developing and had the dialogue continued, I feel confident that she and I together could have made her transition to the unit harmonious. As I was creating this connection, however, another staff member strode forward and stood right in front of her. He said, "That's enough." He shoved the hospital pajamas into her hands and said, "Now take your clothes off and put these on." Paula said, "Don't you talk to me like that." He pointed at her and told her to get in her room and change her clothes. She said, "Don't you point your finger at me. I'm not taking my clothes off."

As the conversation went on, Paula's anger escalated until the staff member pushed her into her room and locked the door. After he left, I looked into the room to see Paula sitting on her bed, with her clothes on, reading her book. A staff member standing nearby commented, "She obviously has Axis Two traits."

Labeling this patient and treating her violently prevented a harmonious transition to the unit. She was scared and confused about being placed in an environment that seemed like a jail. She needed empathy and information, not labels, diagnoses, and violent treatment. For the rest of this patient's stay on the unit, she sought me out when she wanted to talk with someone. Giving her just a little bit of empathy created the atmosphere of safety she needed to be able to openly share her story and her needs.

Domination Systems of Psychiatric Medicine Support Existing Domination Patterns in Families

As an example of this, a twenty-year-old patient diagnosed with schizophrenia had been refusing to take his antipsychotic medications. When his father (a physician) came for a visit, he was angry because he noticed his son was disorganized and delusional and he thought the hospital staff should be giving his son shots when he refused his oral medications. He demanded that the staff exert greater control over his son.

By contrast, the patient's mother realized that even if the patient was forced to take his medications in the hospital, her son would probably not continue to take the pills upon discharge. Building on the opening provided by the patient's mother, I mentioned to the parents that perhaps they could try other healing modalities their son might be more open to. The father asked "Like what?" I relayed a couple of ideas his son told me he was interested in. To each suggestion, the father said, "That won't work."

I suspect this father's insistence on the single-strategy medication answer reflected his own control needs as both a father and a physician. After all, "success" in both roles has traditionally involved exerting power over. Gaining control over disease or control over an unruly child are the classic "good works" of these domination-based roles. But this insistence on control and a single strategy for gaining that control actually created some of the dynamics in his son that this father was so distressed about. The father's strategy of medicating his son without considering and respecting his son's wishes created resistance, rebellion, and confusion. I noticed that the patient's symptoms of confusion and delusional thinking were worse after he visited with his father.

To begin to create a different outcome, empathy is needed all around. The son needs empathy for his reasons for refusing his medications. The father needs empathy for his desire to be a good father and a good physician and for the difficulty of expanding his definition of success in both arenas. In a system set up to gently challenge relationships of control not only within the unit, but between family members, this son might have a chance to heal. As long as the system is aligned with the same power over strategies that reenforce resistance, health care workers cannot begin to understand how to partner with patients to build their skills at meeting their core needs for safety, for autonomy, for relationships of trust, and for recognition of their own truth.

From "Demand and Control" to "Request and Empathy"—A World of Difference

One evening, I was assigned to care for a woman named Erica who had an eating disorder. When I came into work, she was walking around the unit pushing her IV pump (she needed an IV because her electrolytes were out of balance from throwing up). Her pump was beeping because the battery was low. The Charge Nurse said to me, "Tell her to go into her room and plug her pump in. We'll be glad to put her in restraints if she can't cooperate." When I went to talk with Erica, she appeared angry and criticized everything I said. For instance, when I began to verbally express empathy with something she said, she'd immediately interject: "Don't talk to me like that."

I realized that there was nothing I could say that wouldn't stimulate a defensive reaction from her, so I shut my mouth and just listened. Soon Erica asked, "Why aren't you saying anything?" I replied, "I'm confused because I don't know what I could say that wouldn't piss you off." At that point, her anger toward me dissolved and she became more receptive. I told her I was concerned that her IV would clot off if she didn't plug the IV pump in and asked her if she would be willing to plug it in. She said she would after using the bathroom. The rest of the shift I listened to her with empathy and made requests instead of demands. At the end of the shift she said, "Thanks for being so cool to me. I feel a lot better." She also said that when staff members told her what to do in an unkind way, "It pisses me off," and then she didn't want to do it.

Erica's story is a perfect example of the different results that are possible by shifting from a "demand and control" communication pattern to a "request and empathy" model of NVC. Using empathy and making respectful requests to patients is much more likely to elicit cooperation than using judgments, analyses, and making demands. Why? The answer is simple. You cannot make anyone do anything. Yes, you can use force to make someone regret they didn't do what you wanted; but if you want someone to act in a beneficial way toward themselves and toward others, communication is the key.

Are You Demanding or Requesting?

Understanding how your own habitual communication style perpetuates dysfunctional patterns of behavior in others is the first step in learning how to communicate in a way that creates win-win solutions. Using power over tactics and making demands perpetuates patient's habitual patterns of reactivity. Using empathy and making requests instead of demands creates the foundation of human connection which makes it possible for everyone to have their needs met. Let's explore in greater detail the difference between requests and demands and trace the ways in which these different communication methods create very different results.

Every time you demand something of a patient, you trigger their autonomy and control issues. The human desire for autonomy and self-determination is so powerful that patients will resist demands even if it means harming themselves. Erica, for example, had already proved that you couldn't make her eat. She had been proving it for twenty-five years. No doubt the need for a sense of control was itself a significant factor in sustaining her eating disorder. Why would anyone expect her to submit quietly to external demands and control tactics? What if, instead, you viewed Erica's passionate drive for self-control as a potential key element in her recovery? Only by treating her with compassion and respect can you we begin to unlock her autonomy dynamics in ways that might be healing.

Patients are not the only ones who have strong needs for self-control. Just as patients will choose self-damaging behavior over submissive behavior, so will many staff members. Your need for autonomy is often greater than your desire to keep your job or to stay on the "good side" of a Charge Nurse who exploits her power. Many a staff member has chosen to walk away rather than submit to a demand they view as arbitrary or in violation of their fundamental right to self-determination.

How Can You Tell a Demand From a Request?

On the surface, the difference between a demand and a request may seem simple. A request provides choice; a demand does not. "Would you please put on your shoes" sounds like a request; "Put your shoes on now" is clearly a demand.

Some demands, however, are trickier to spot because they are disguised as requests. The best way to judge the difference is to look at the consequences attached to the choice. If a request is made and a "No" answer triggers punishment, the request was never a request at all, but a demand in disguise. Here's an example: If I ask a patient "Would you please put on your shoes," and my patient says "No," then what? If my response is to punish the patient verbally, physically, or by withdrawing something they value, I can be sure that my request was actually a demand. If my question "Would you please put on your shoes," was truly a request, when the patient responded with "No," she would have received understanding, not punishment.

Demands masquerading as requests are common in nursing cultures, too. If a Charge Nurse asks you to do something and you elect not to do it, it is likely that punishment of some kind will follow. The problem is that demands funnel the recipient into an impossible dilemma, either give in to the demand by saying "Yes," or be punished for saying "No." You can either submit or rebel. If you submit, you'll feel resentful because to do so goes against your needs for autonomy and respect. And the more you don't honor your needs—especially for autonomy and respect—the more likely it is that you'll suffer burnout.

Practicing the art of making true requests—that is, offering real choices with compassion and acceptance of either the yes or the no response—is a critical strategy for creating safe environments. All humans have a fundamental need for self-control and autonomy. If you honor that need and work with it instead of against it, you can stop triggering the resistance and rebellion that is a natural effect of the power over system.

The Pervasiveness of Violence and the Need to Heal Yourself

Moving from power over to power with communication patterns is a key part of a shift toward safe, nonviolent healing environments for people with psychiatric illnesses. It is important to notice, however, that psychiatric medicine is practiced in the context of a culture that celebrates violence. The larger task of intervening in that violence requires you to acknowledge fully the violence that pervades your culture and your own lives. And you cannot do that without looking carefully within yourself.

You must begin by acknowledging that the United States is one of the most violent countries in the world. You are socialized to be violent—through cartoons, movies, video games, and the judgmental language you speak. You use words about others such as right and wrong, good and bad, attractive and unattractive, competent and incompetent; terms which can stimulate pain and frustration. These concepts are so ingrained in your consciousness that you are blinded to the violence of them. For example—you use the word *deserve* to justify punishing and rewarding people. If someone does what you like, "They deserve to be rewarded." If someone doesn't do what you want, "They deserve to be punished." With the word *deserve*, you become the judge and executioner of others.

In 1971, a study was done called the Stanford Prison Experiment. In that study, normal college students were randomly assigned to play the role of guard or inmate for two weeks in a simulated prison, yet the guards quickly became so brutal that the experiment had to be shut down after only six days. Whenever one group of people dominates another, violence is likely.

If you are to successfully end the violence in health care organizations, you must begin by investigating your own wounded-ness as well as your capacity to become—like the Stanford "guards"—unwitting pawns of the dynamics of a domination system. To change the violence outside of you, you must first change the violence within yourself. This means inquiring compassionately into your own experiences as both victims and perpetrators of violence. Identifying violence in others is not difficult, but many of you don't wake up to your own capacity for violence until something dramatic happens. However, until you consciously own your own violence, you will unconsciously project it onto others.

The truth is that without the proper support and tools to overcome culturally conditioned patterns of reacting violently to frustrating situations, anyone can become violent. Each employee's unresolved orientation toward violence—combined with a language that dehumanizes people by labeling them—helps create and maintain an abusive environment. Employees who project their own violence onto patients are likely to treat patients in hostile, aggressive, and violent ways, striking out at those who seem threatening and becoming verbally aggressive when they don't get their way.

Even the most dedicated staff member can become frustrated working day in and day out with patients who can be angry, hostile, and violent and who sometimes actively resist the care the staff are working so hard to provide. In such volatile environments, it is easy to vent one's frustration by abusing or striking out at a patient. Without deliberate efforts to address each individual employee's personal relationship to violence, the dynamics of psychiatric units will continue to set the stage for perpetuating the violence cycle.

Acknowledging the Effects of Childhood Abuse

Changing habitual patterns is a healing process. As Albert Einstein says, "We cannot solve problems by using the same kind of thinking we used when we created them." Shifting to a new kind of thinking is precisely what the tools of NVC are about. By using the tools of

NVC, you find yourself experiencing a different consciousness and from this new way of thinking, you can discover ways to stop the violence and heal yourself and others. You can also use the language of NVC to create different systems that are based on your current values, not on unconscious habitual programming.

Changing your patterns begins with awareness, and awareness takes courage and support. The truth is that unless you take a hard look at violence toward children in the culture, you will never successfully intervene in a meaningful way into the cycle of violence in psychiatric units and health care organizations more generally.

Often, when children grow up in an abusive household, they identify with the oppressor, believe they are being punished for their own good and justify their own abusive behavior later in life. They say things like, "I was spanked and it didn't harm me. I turned out OK." For instance, parents will perpetuate the abuse they suffered as children onto their own children until they become aware of what was done to them and experience the feelings and needs that they repressed.

Similarly, when these abused children—still unaware of their repressed feelings—grow up and begin working in a psychiatric unit, they believe that they are helping patients by putting them in restraints or using other punitive measures. They believe they are teaching them how to behave in the world just like they were taught to behave when they were children.

A fascinating insight for all healing professions is another way in which childhood abuse manifests its effects later in life. When you are not aware of the abuse that happened to you as a child, it will often express itself in your body in the form of illness. According to Christiane Northrup, M.D., every emotion is a biochemical reality in the body. Emotions that are repressed express themselves physically. When you allow yourself to feel these emotions and learn the truth about your history, then physical healing can occur.

Learning the truth and telling the truth can take tremendous courage. Your healing, and your patients' healing, requires you to move beyond cultural norms and risk feeling things that go against some deeply ingrained beliefs. In her book, *The Body Never Lies*, for example,

Alice Miller describes a woman who had uterine cancer. In order to heal her cancer, this woman had to acknowledge that her parents abused her as a child. To speak this personal truth required her to go against the powerful cultural edict to love, honor, and obey your parents. Once she risked telling her truth and experienced her repressed feelings about what had happened, the cancer went away.

My own history provides another example of how unresolved childhood violence is carried forward into all one's relationships. My parents raised me in a way that was accepted and normal in this culture. They thought they were doing me a favor by judging, criticizing, shaming, and spanking me as I grew up. They wanted me to be able to survive in the world. But the results of that upbringing were the opposite of what they wanted. The damage to my self-esteem and confidence made it more difficult for me to survive. In order to survive in a healthy way, I had to find my own path back to empathy and compassion.

As someone who has experienced the long term effects of verbal, emotional, and physical abuse and also experienced the effect of being treated with empathy and compassion, it is clear to me which treatment is effective in producing happy, well-adjusted, confident people who can contribute to society.

Part of healing yourself is about learning to see the humanity in others, no matter how they behave. Holding on to blame keeps you stuck in victim consciousness. Although it is important to understand what happened to you growing up and receive empathy for unresolved pain, it is also important to eventually understand the needs your parents were meeting and not meeting when they acted in a manner that was hurtful to you. As long as you think in terms of right and wrong and hold onto labels of others, you will not be able to own unconscious parts of yourself.

How Will You End the Cycle of Violence?

In this chapter, you've looked at a number of ways to intervene in the violent legacy of psychiatric medicine. Some of the work is individual. You are each responsible for understanding your personal relationships to violence as victims and as perpetrators within your socially sanctioned domination systems. You can each do the very personal work of seeking resolution and healing the wounds left from childhood violence and become very intentional about not repeating those patterns in your own families or in your work as health care professionals.

As individuals, you also have the power to learn new communication skills. You can become aware of the difference between a demand and a request and you can practice empathy every chance you get with yourself, your colleagues, your patients, and the families with whom you partner to find successful strategies of healing for mental illness.

Creating nonviolent models of psychiatric medicine also calls you to tackle systems-level issues. You must challenge some foundational beliefs about mental illness and have the courage to break out of your single-minded focus on individual physiology. This means challenging some of the basic assumptions feeding your enormous pharmaceutical industry as well.

Ultimately, you must become more interested in positive results for people with mental illness. Your desire to support real healing and create fewer broken lives must be stronger than your desire to control and dominate. NVC teaches you that this is not just a pipe dream. There are specific skills that can create the partnership relationships necessary to support healing. When you champion those skills in health care organizations, your families, and yourself, you can begin to build a less violent world.

Notes: _____

1. Martin Buber, Buber, *Between Man and Man* (New York: Routledge Classics, 2002), p. xii.

Chapter 6

Compassion, Empathy, and Honesty: A Road Map for Creating Life-serving Systems of Care

Coming Alive at Work

find it tragic that people spend their lives working at jobs that are repressive and do not meet their human needs. When I was a hospice nurse, I got the message that life is precious and is to be lived fully. Since then, I have been on a mission to do what contributes to making me feel alive.

> Don't ask yourself what the world needs;
> Ask yourself what makes you come alive.
> And then go and do that.
> Because what the world needs
> Is people who have come alive.[1]

Health care systems have tremendous potential for creating life-serving systems. The people who work in health care are enormously caring, dedicated, and hard-working. There's no question that with the right tools, these educated professionals can create healing environments for themselves and their patients.

However, when these same caring and skilled individuals find themselves caught up in some of the systems discussed here, the results are more damaging than healing—a state of affairs which is enormously painful for health care workers and the patients who depend on them for care. Using the tools of Nonviolent Communication (NVC), you can create organizations that nurture rather than stifle life energy; strong, humane places in which people flourish. In such organizations, great teams work together to provide care for patients. Individuals are celebrated for their uniqueness, and empathy and support flow. Communications are open so that problems are addressed and healing occurs. You can create organizations that truly deliver life-serving systems of care.

In earlier chapters, I've spoken extensively about how compassion and empathy have the power to transform your relationships to one another and to your patients. As you turn to the practical question of how to bring those and other NVC principles into the culture of your organization, it is important to take a hard look at a third dimension of NVC: Honesty. Without a foundation of honesty, you cannot begin to build successful partnerships with yourself, your colleagues, your organizations, and your patients. Without a foundational expectation of truth-telling, even the best road map cannot help you travel away from the domination model and toward the partnership model of communication and care.

What Does Dishonesty Have to Do With Aliveness?

In the domination model which most of you were raised in, you were socialized to be dishonest. You learned that it is "not nice" to express your honesty toward others, especially if they are suffering, so you stuff your truth along with your feelings and become nice dead people. Fearing that your wants and needs might be in conflict with the wants and needs of others, you believe you are doing someone a favor by not expressing your truth. As a result, you go through life with painted smiles when underneath you are crying to be seen and understood. The epidemic of depression is a symptom of this. Despite the high costs of this version of "niceness," you come to believe that your social lives depend on it. You believe that telling the truth will cost you the acceptance of your peers—your very worst fear. So, you perpetuate the behavior of dishonesty, and this choice makes healthy partnership relationships almost impossible to sustain.

Dishonesty Creates Disconnection and Perpetuates Delusional Thinking

It is difficult to connect with someone who is not telling the truth about how he or she feels. And, in the absence of real information about the truth of someone's feelings, it is very hard to clear up misperceptions and come to a shared picture of reality.

I learned that a patient of mine had built up a romantic fantasy about a staff worker. I suggested that it would be useful to orient the patient to reality, and proposed to have the patient talk to the staff member about his fantasy and then have the staff member express her truth to the patient. Upon hearing this, several staff members said, "We cannot do that, he's sick and has already had a hard day." But the truth, even though hard to hear, might have made the patient's tomorrow easier. We all, generally, like to know the truth—even when it initially hurts.

Sympathy and pity often prevent honesty from occurring. However, the more you protect others from having hurt feelings, the more you enable them to continue seeing the world in a delusional way. Honesty is a gift to others, even if it doesn't feel like it in the moment. Sometimes suffering—the very suffering you lie to protect others from—is necessary in order to break down illusions and create the kind of perception-shift that opens up new worlds of possibility. You cannot live an authentic life unless you are willing to be honest and are willing to receive another's honesty.

Honesty Can Trigger Blame, Which Is the Projection of a Wish for Empathy

Many people react negatively when they hear honesty and will blame and judge you. That's how you're conditioned to deal with pain. In many cultures, when life is full of pain you look for someone to blame. Instead of using the painful stimulus as an opportunity to own your feelings, you project them onto others in the form of blame, criticism, or judgment.

When you, as health care workers, don't understand this dynamic, taking care of sick people can become a minefield. Inevitably, you step on a mine, because you become a convenient target for others' disowned pain. Even if you have perfect clinical and interpersonal skills, you'll become the target for patients and families as they unconsciously try to get empathy. If you understand that people ask for empathy by expressing blame, you have a better chance of meeting their needs and not taking it personally.

Specific Ways to Express Honesty

There are various levels of honesty. You can be honest about your judgments, although if you communicate them verbally, you can expect a defensive reaction from others. If you recognize that another person's actions are the stimulus and not the cause of your feelings, you can take ownership of your judgments, realize they are about you, and express your judgments in terms of your own feelings and needs. To communicate in this way is to change from an outward focus of expressing yourself to an inward one and is more likely to elicit cooperation from others. Using the steps of NVC, you can express your honesty using the four steps of the model: observations, feelings, needs, and requests.

Take the example: "Mary is a rude person" (this is an outwardly focused judgment). If you say to Mary, "You are a rude person," you're very likely to stimulate Mary into a defensive reaction. You can, however, express your honesty in another way—one that's a lot less likely to trigger someone's defenses and a lot more likely to open up communication.

The NVC model for that looks like this: "When you spoke at the meeting before I'd finished speaking [Observation], I felt frustrated [Feeling], because I really wanted my point of view to be understood. [Need], Can you tell me what you're hearing me say?" [Request]

Expressing your honesty in this form will open up communication. Even if Mary has a defensive reaction, you can use the NVC tools to help create a connection. For instance, if Mary says, "You are not the only one with something important to say," you can respond by giving her empathy; this would sound like:

"Were you feeling anxious [Feeling] because you needed to be heard and recognized for your contribution?" [Need]

Or instead of giving her empathy, you can ask her again to listen to your message.

NVC teaches that you are responsible for how you communicate and for your own intentions. You are not responsible for how others receive your messages. You can be responsive to others' reactions, but you are not responsible for them.

When you don't express your honesty to those you work with, the environment becomes cluttered with misunderstandings and disconnections. Without a bedrock of honest communication, your own assumptions cloud how you view others and you develop enemy images. Functional teams cannot be built and going to work is about as much fun as having a migraine headache.

Expressing Honesty in the Face of Authority

In hierarchical systems, the cost of honesty can seem especially high. Nurses, for example, are often afraid to be honest with those in authority. They fear losing their job, so they complain to their co-workers about problems on the unit and feel angry and resentful. One evening during a unit meeting with the Nursing Director, I expressed my feelings of anxiety when I was assigned to be the medication nurse because I feared being punished if I made a mistake. This opened up a dialogue as other nurses also tentatively expressed their concerns with the current medication system. At one point the Nursing Director said, "If people aren't honest with me about their feelings, what am I supposed to do?"

After the meeting, I ran into the Director in the hall and told her that I did not have a problem with her personally but that I needed to express my feelings about issues that adversely affected me. Before I could say anything else, she glanced at me with a look that I interpreted as angry and, without saying anything, turned her back and walked away.

I imagined that she felt hurt and wanted recognition and appreciation for the job she did—but the way that she communicated this made me doubt that she cared about hearing people's honesty. I understood why staff members were afraid to be honest with her.

Other staff members thanked me for speaking up and several of them said they were too frightened to speak up as I did. Everyone was aware of the issue but no one had dared to bring it up. This fear of being honest is indigenous to the culture. It occurs not only in workplaces but also in intimate relationships, in families, and in most group situations.

Honesty Can Be Risky, But Dishonesty Is Always Riskier

Honesty creates intimacy and connection. It also helps organizations become aware of issues and implement changes that create more safety for patients, and less stress for staff. So, why don't people express the truth more often in organizations? One reason is that people fear their honesty will stir up problems they won't be able to resolve. Since studying NVC, I can express my honesty because I'm confident I have the tools to clean up any mess I create. I'm also willing to risk losing my job because I know that when I don't express my honesty, I lose more than that: I lose my self-respect. As I have become more aware of my needs, I have become smarter about when I choose to express honesty and when to remain quiet. Until systems support honest open communication, it will be risky to express honesty about certain things.

Organizations lose, too, when dishonesty is perpetuated as a cultural norm. Administrators don't know which systems are ineffective not only because staff refuse to express their honesty about how systems affect them, but also because staff members actually lie about their issues. Nurses I've worked with in a variety of settings tell the people in charge what they think they want to hear instead of what's true. This perpetuates the delusional outlook administrators sometimes maintain, and permits ineffective systems to continue adversely affecting employees and patients.

One staff member on my unit told the administrator he was fine with an issue he'd told me he was in a lot of pain about. At another place I worked, a survey asked employees to give honest feedback about their managers and assured them they wouldn't be punished for telling the truth. Even though many of the employees told me they hated a certain manager and complained about him daily, on the survey they praised him. Unless people are willing to tell the truth, the system will stay the same and people will continue to feel angry and frustrated because their needs are not being met.

These lies and withholdings of truth may seem small or petty, but the consequences can be catastrophic. A few years ago, a hospital was in the news because a patient died just outside of the Emergency Room. The staff knew the patient was there but because the hospital policy did not allow treatment at that location, the patient was left to die. I suspect that the hospital would have appreciated it if someone had questioned that policy and acted to save that person's life, thus avoiding the public relations outcry that occurred in the community.

Building Organizations That Consider Everyone's Needs Requires Honest Communication Without Fear of Reprisal

To change this ingrained behavior of dishonesty, employers need to create a safe space where employees can practice being honest and can receive empathy for what gets stirred up by doing so. Using the tools of NVC, they can begin to change habitual patterns of dishonesty and use the NVC model as a guideline for expressing their honesty.

Honoring employees and encouraging them to express the truth and even to disagree with those in power goes a long way toward assuring them that their opinions are respected. When an employee openly and without fear of reprisal shares with a supervisor information about the needs that cannot be met by complying with a request, the supervisor learns not only how to better meet the needs of that employee but also discovers how to support that employee so he or she can better do their job. Making demands is a normal part of the operating procedure in a bureaucratic system. Institutions that demand blind obedience to authority and punish nonconformity are adversely affected by their own policies.

Ten Starter-ideas for Integrating NVC Into Your Organization

There are many different steps you can take to bring the insights of NVC into your organization. Below are some ideas for how to begin.

1. Evaluate your systems. Which ones can be changed from "power over" systems to "power with" systems? Is your overall organization a hierarchal system? If so, you may want to explore other successful and efficient forms of organization such as Sociocracy. Sociocracy is a form of management that presumes equality of individuals and is based on consent. It encourages open communication and inclusion of all staff in the decision-making process.

2. Create an emotionally safe environment. There are a number of ways to create a culture that acknowledges and supports honest expression of feelings and needs. Managers can be taught how to listen from the heart using the NVC model of empathy. Even staff evaluations can become a tool that opens up communication. One way to do this is to have staff do a self-evaluation and sit down with their manager and discuss it. The manager can voice any concerns she or he may have after she has listened clearly and fully to the staff. Then the staff person can

listen to the manager's concerns and can respond to that. Having a mediator present that understands how to use NVC to mediate conflict would be very valuable in this process.

3. Encourage staff to participate in making decisions that affect their work. Routinely enrolling staff in decision-making and strategy setting is a key element in creating a system that values all members and all perspectives. The process of co-creating policies and processes helps staff connect with one another and gives them a personal stake in implementing mutually agreed-upon strategies. In a partnership framework, it seems very clear that the people who do the work know what can be done to make things easier and safer better than the manager who does not do the work.

4. Build in routine time for NVC check-in. Include a time to connect during report at the beginning and end of each shift. This could be a brief check-in for the nurses or a time to discuss a NVC concept and solicit ideas of how to implement that concept. For instance, the check-in facilitator might solicit examples from the staff about how and when they can make use of a specific NVC concept, such as "Empathy Before Education."

An idea for a check-in (or a check-out for the nurses who have just worked) would be to express something they did during their shift that they feel happy about and also something that they feel stressed about. For instance a nurse could say, "I was able to verbally de-escalate my patient by using NVC. This prevented him from being placed in restraints and it helped me feel more confident with my skills." She can go on to say, "I feel sad because I was hoping to help my other patient take a shower and I didn't have time. He hasn't had a shower for a week and his hair is filthy."

Similarly, staff coming on might state anything they feel stressed about, any fears or regrets left over from previous shifts, or any hopes they have for the shift. This kind of vulnerable sharing will only work once staff members feel safe sharing. Assuring people that they won't be judged, analyzed, or put down if they share honestly and demonstrating that anything they say will be received with empathy will go a long way in creating emotional safety. This kind of honest and vulnerable sharing will create community and caring between staff members. This will allow them to work together in a productive and harmonious way.

5. Whenever a stressful situation happens, take a few minutes to debrief. Use NVC to empathize with the feelings and reactions in the staff that got stimulated by the situation. Discuss ways to use NVC to prevent such a situation from occurring again.

6. Schedule a staff person with advanced empathy skills on each shift. If something difficult happens, that person would be available to give empathy to people who need it. Nurses or other staff members can ask for empathy if they feel scared after a dangerous event or if they get hurt on the job. People can use the identified empathy person to help them resolve conflicts or to help them express something that may be difficult to express.

6. Educate staff about NVC. Give laminated NVC process cards for easy, ongoing reference. Put charts up on the wall. Refer to the charts when debriefing or during report. Make the language and principles of NVC part of the everyday culture of your team.

7. Think of training as an ongoing process, not a one-time event. NVC is something to practice over time. Instituting regular training sessions in NVC will allow staff to advance their skills and talk about the challenges they may be having using the tools. It is not easy to change the way you communicate. It takes intention, support, and practice.

8. In the psychiatric unit, all patients need a de-escalating plan. Patients can help staff write the plan. Patients can explain what they do when they start to get upset (i.e., pacing, speaking loudly, cussing, overeating) and they can identify what calms them down (music, empathy, warm baths, private time, etc.) For those patients with less than optimal cognitive function, staff members can try and anticipate the patient's needs when they see them become upset. Since all people have the same needs, giving empathy to all patients and trying strategies to help meet needs will help create a safe unit.

9. Create an expectation that employees will address their concerns directly with the person they have an issue with. Supporting this expectation with skill-building training and recognition for success will

decrease gossip and clear up misunderstandings. Someone skilled in NVC can act as a mediator for hard-to-discuss issues.

10. Create a code phrase to trigger an intervention in violent or toxic staff communication behaviors. At Mendota Mental Health Institute in Wisconsin, the Maximum Treatment Unit has instituted a system that allows intervention when a staff person notices "toxic" behavior from a fellow staff member toward a patient. The staff person says, "You have a phone call." Then the person who is acting in a way that is less than therapeutic goes into the office where she/he can get empathy in private. When a staff member is acting nontherapeutically with a patient, it is a sign that they are stressed. When they get empathy, they will feel supported and their emotional energy will change so that they will be more able to deal with patients in a compassionate way. This kind of ongoing empathy will also help staff grow emotionally and will integrate the tools of NVC. NVC is best learned from experiencing it emotionally. If you only understand the concepts intellectually, it will be very difficult if not impossible to be able to use them when you need them.

These are just a few of the millions of creative strategies you might invent to implement NVC into your health care program. Since your program is unique, you will need to devise unique strategies. What makes sense for your program? Building a safe and nurturing environment for both patients and staff will be an enriching journey for all involved.

Life-serving Organizations Meet Everyone's Needs

One evening, upon arriving for work, I walked past a too-common scene in the hallway. A nurse was standing in the hallway outside a patient's door, yelling the repeated demand "Go sit on your bed!" Meanwhile, the patient was banging on the other side of the door and insisting that she wanted to come out. The situation appeared to be locked in a classic stalemate born of unmet control needs.

I looked in the small cell-like window and said, "Hi Mary, go sit on your bed. I want to come in and talk with you." When Mary saw me, her face lit up and she ran over and sat on her bed. The nurse standing at the door said, "That's amazing. How did you do that?" I had no magic potion, no pills or tricks. However, I had worked with the patient the week before and, using the tools of NVC, had created a nurturing connection with her. The patient was not willing to submit to the demands of a staff member with whom she did not feel a connection, yet she cooperated willingly when treated with respect and compassion.

Empathy is one of the simplest yet most potent human technologies on the planet. It is a low-cost, high-yield solution that everyone can use. Most of all, it is nothing you need to "add" to your systems, it is already part of who you are as human beings. It is your birthright, if only you can create organizations that support you in using your humanity as a tool for connection and healing.

In the Maximum Treatment Unit at Mendota Mental Health Institute, both the staff and the patients take classes in NVC. They have created a sanctuary there that promotes recovery. Since implementing NVC in their unit, the culture of the unit has changed from one of violence to one of peace and harmony. Staff turnover and staff injuries have stopped and nurses are now competing to work on the unit that used to be one of the worst places to work. The patients are actually getting better and are being transferred to less restrictive units. Patients and staff say, "It's safe now."

The unit has become a life-serving system. Don't you all deserve to work and receive care in equally safe and healing places?

Throughout this book, you've explored how the "empathy tool" of NVC expands your ability to listen to the hearts of others and how potentially violent situations can be transformed into caring connections. You've seen that it is possible to create systems that provide harmony and serve you at all levels. It is clear that your patients, your staff members, and your organizations all benefit when you turn your language and your systems in the direction of partnership and care.

Hurtful systems of blame, scapegoating, reward, punishment, power over, and backstabbing are not inevitable or "natural." You do not need to stand for them or live with the damage they do to your spirits, your bodies, and your minds. If you are willing to open your minds and hearts, you can shift your perception and see how these negative patterns are actually symptoms of larger systems of domination: systems which feed on judgments, disconnection, and untruths.

Hospitals need workers who are willing to speak out against policies that are incongruent with their life-serving mission. They must recognize that their employees are human beings with human needs. If those needs are not acknowledged and respected, the hospital will struggle with personnel issues, and quality of care will continue to suffer.

As you turn in the direction of partnership and honor the feelings and needs that make you human, you can evolve life-serving organizations in which care and healing are supported at every level. You can meet one another's deepest needs for understanding and respect. And, in the process, you can save countless dollars now spent on replacing burnt-out workers and resolving medical mistakes linked to broken processes no one will talk about and judgment errors stemming from lack of empathy.

As health care evolves, the underlying belief systems and mode of communication also need to change. NVC provides the tools you need to rebuild your relationships and rethink the systems and processes that support your safety, growth, and learning. The time is now to pick up these tools and get to work. I envision a nurturing workplace where health care workers can serve their fellow human beings with open hearts. It is a workplace that is fun, supportive, and life-affirming. Won't you join me? There is so much to heal and so little to lose.

Notes: _____

1. Harold Whitman, "Motivational Quotes and Quotations."
   www.bestmotivation.com/quotes-1/of/Harold_Whitman.htm

Index

A

abandoned, as pseudo-feeling, 14–15

abused, as pseudo-feeling, 7, 14–15

action-oriented requests, 8–9

active listening versus empathy, 12–13

acupuncture, 26

advice giving, as communication block, 13–14, 55

affection, as human need, 8

analysis, as dysfunctional communication pattern, 6–8, 13–14, 29–32, 50–54

anger, empathy to diffuse, 15

appropriate/inappropriate paradigm, 35

attacked, as pseudo-feeling, 7

authenticity, in partnership systems, 35

authority figures in domination systems, 24–27, 51–54, 67–68

autonomy needs, 24–25, 69–71

B

backstabbing, as dysfunctional communication, 43, 45, 88–89

bad/good paradigm, 24, 35, 71–72

behavior, as attempt to meet needs, 62, 65

belief, impact on healing and disease, 52–54. *See also* self-fulfilling prophecy, judgments as

betrayed, as pseudo-feeling, 7

blame, as dysfunctional communication pattern, 6–8, 29–34, 41–43, 74, 80, 88–89

The Body Never Lies (Miller), 73–74

Buber, Martin, 63

bullied, as pseudo-feeling, 14–15

burden, needs as, 11–12

burnout rate of hospice nurses. *See also* self-fulfilling prophecy, judgments as

business, evolution from domination-based to partnership model, 22–23

C

calming effect of empathy, 14

caring, devaluation in domination systems, 25–26, 35

cheapness of life, in domination systems, 35

cheated, as pseudo-feeling, 14–15

check-in, with NVC, 85

child abuse, effects of, 72–74

child/parent relationships, evolution from domination to partnership model, 21–22, 24, 73–74

choice, as prerequisite for change, 64

choice-making with children, 22

choices, personal responsibility for, 9–10

co-creation of policies with staff, 85

code phrase to trigger staff intervention, 87

communication patterns, as belief systems perpetuated through language, 6, 29–32

The Four-Part Nonviolent Communication Process

Clearly expressing	Empathically receiving
how **I am**	how **you are**
without blaming	without hearing
or criticizing	blame or criticism

OBSERVATIONS

1. What I observe *(see, hear, remember, imagine, free from my evaluations)* that does or does not contribute to my well-being:

   "When I (see, hear) . . . "

1. What you observe *(see, hear, remember, imagine, free from your evaluations)* that does or does not contribute to your well-being:

   "When you see/hear . . . "

   (Sometimes unspoken when offering empathy)

FEELINGS

2. How I feel *(emotion or sensation rather than thought)* in relation to what I observe:

   "I feel . . . "

2. How you feel *(emotion or sensation rather than thought)* in relation to what you observe:

   "You feel . . . "

NEEDS

3. What I need or value *(rather than a preference, or a specific action)* that causes my feelings:

   " . . . because I need/value . . . "

3. What you need or value *(rather than a preference, or a specific action)* that causes your feelings:

   " . . . because you need/value . . . "

Clearly requesting that	Empathically receiving that
which would enrich **my**	which would enrich **your** life
life without demanding	without hearing any demand

REQUESTS

4. The concrete actions I would like taken:

   "Would you be willing to . . . ?"

4. The concrete actions you would like taken:

   "Would you like . . . ?"

   (Sometimes unspoken when offering empathy)

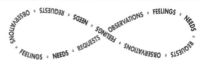

Some Basic Feelings We All Have

Feelings when needs are fulfilled

- Amazed
- Comfortable
- Confident
- Eager
- Energetic
- Fulfilled
- Glad
- Hopeful
- Inspired
- Intrigued
- Joyous
- Moved
- Optimistic
- Proud
- Relieved
- Stimulated
- Surprised
- Thankful
- Touched
- Trustful

Feelings when needs are not fulfilled

- Angry
- Annoyed
- Concerned
- Confused
- Disappointed
- Discouraged
- Distressed
- Embarrassed
- Frustrated
- Helpless
- Hopeless
- Impatient
- Irritated
- Lonely
- Nervous
- Overwhelmed
- Puzzled
- Reluctant
- Sad
- Uncomfortable

Some Basic Needs We All Have

Autonomy
- Choosing dreams/goals/values
- Choosing plans for fulfilling one's dreams, goals, values

Celebration
- Celebrating the creation of life and dreams fulfilled
- Celebrating losses: loved ones, dreams, etc. (mourning)

Integrity
- Authenticity • Creativity
- Meaning • Self-worth

Interdependence
- Acceptance • Appreciation
- Closeness • Community
- Consideration
- Contribution to the enrichment of life
- Emotional Safety • Empathy

Physical Nurturance
- Air • Food
- Movement, exercise
- Protection from life-threatening forms of life: viruses, bacteria, insects, predatory animals
- Rest • Sexual Expression
- Shelter • Touch • Water

Play
- Fun • Laughter

Spiritual Communion
- Beauty • Harmony
- Inspiration • Order • Peace

- Honesty (the empowering honesty that enables us to learn from our limitations)
- Love • Reassurance
- Respect • Support
- Trust • Understanding

About PuddleDancer Press

PuddleDancer Press (PDP) is the premier publisher of Nonviolent Communication™ related works. Its mission is to provide high-quality materials to help people create a world in which all needs are met compassionately. Publishing revenues are used to develop new books, and implement promotion campaigns for NVC and Marshall Rosenberg. By working in partnership with the Center for Nonviolent Communication and NVC trainers, teams, and local supporters, PDP has created a comprehensive promotion effort that has helped bring NVC to thousands of new people each year.

Since 2003 PDP has donated more than 60,000 NVC books to organizations, decision-makers, and individuals in need around the world. This program is supported in part by donations made to CNVC and by partnerships with like-minded organizations around the world. PDP is a core partner of the Help Share NVC Project, giving access to hundreds of valuable tools, resources, and ideas to help NVC trainers and supporters make NVC a household name by creating financially sustainable training practices. Learn more at www.helpsharenvc.com.

Visit the PDP website at www.NonviolentCommunication.com to find the following resources:

- **Shop NVC**—Continue your learning. Purchase our NVC titles online safely, affordably, and conveniently. Find everyday discounts on individual titles, multiple-copies, and book packages. Learn more about our authors and read endorsements of NVC from world-renowned communication experts and peacemakers.

- **NVC Quick Connect e-Newsletter**—Sign up today to receive our monthly e-Newsletter, filled with expert articles, upcoming training opportunities with our authors, and exclusive specials on NVC learning materials. Archived e-Newsletters are also available

- **About NVC**—Learn more about these life-changing communication and conflict resolution skills including an overview of the NVC process, key facts about NVC, and more.

- **About Marshall Rosenberg**—Access press materials, biography, and more about this world-renowned peacemaker, educator, bestselling author, and founder of the Center for Nonviolent Communication.

- **Free Resources for Learning NVC**—Find free weekly tips series, NVC article archive, and other great resources to make learning these vital communication skills just a little easier.

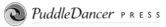

For more information, please contact PuddleDancer Press at:

2240 Encinitas Blvd., Ste. D-911 • Encinitas, CA 92024
Phone: 858-759-6963 • Fax: 858-759-6967
Email: email@puddledancer.com • www.NonviolentCommunication.com

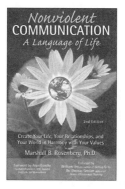

Nonviolent Communication:
A Language of Life, Second Edition

Create Your Life, Your Relationships, and Your World in Harmony With Your Values

Marshall B. Rosenberg, Ph.D.

$19.95 — Trade Paper 6x9, 240pp
ISBN: 978-1-892005-03-8

In this internationally acclaimed text, Marshall Rosenberg offers insightful stories, anecdotes, practical exercises and role-plays that will literally change your approach to communication for the better. Nonviolent Communication partners practical skills with a powerful consciousness to help us get what we want peacefully.

Discover how the language you use can strengthen your relationships, build trust, prevent or resolve conflicts peacefully, and heal pain. More than 400,000 copies of this landmark text have been sold in twenty languages around the globe.

"Nonviolent Communication is a simple yet powerful methodology for communicating in a way that meets both parties' needs. This is one of the most useful books you will ever read."

—**William Ury**, coauthor of *Getting to Yes* and author of *The Third Side*

"I believe the principles and techniques in this book can literally change the world, but more importantly, they can change the quality of your life with your spouse, your children, your neighbors, your co-workers, and everyone else you interact with."

—**Jack Canfield**, author, *Chicken Soup for the Soul*

SAVE 10% at NonviolentCommunication.com with coupon code: **bookads**

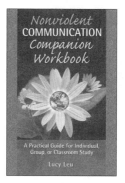

Nonviolent Communication Companion Workbook

A Practical Guide for Individual, Group, or Classroom Study

by Lucy Leu

$21.95 — Trade Paper 7x10, 224pp
ISBN: 978-1-892005-04-5

Learning Nonviolent Communication has often been equated with learning a whole new language. The *NVC Companion Workbook* helps you put these powerful, effective skills into practice with chapter-by-chapter study of Marshall Rosenberg's cornerstone text, *NVC: A Language of Life*. Create a safe, supportive group learning or practice environment that nurtures the needs of each participant. Find a wealth of activities, exercises, and facilitator suggestions to refine and practice this powerful communication process.

Available from PuddleDancer Press, the Center for Nonviolent Communication, all major bookstores, and Amazon.com. Distributed by Independent Publisher's Group: 800-888-4741.

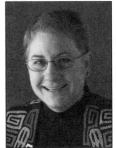

Photo by John Cornicello

Melanie Sears, RN, MBA, has been a CNVC certified trainer since 1991. She works with businesses, hospitals, nursing homes, hospices, individuals, couples, and parents in transforming communication and interactions to ones that are more compassionate, conscious, and effective.

Melanie presents Nonviolent Communication at conventions, at universities, and at churches. She has been interviewed on the radio and on television, and is the author of several titles, including the workbook *Choose Your Words: Harnessing the Power of Compassionate Communication to Heal and Connect* available at **www.dnadialogues.com**. Her presentations have been described as exciting, inspiring, educational, and transformative.

Melanie says, "Everything is about communications. Any problem can be resolved within minutes when negative energy is transformed into caring connections."

Melanie has worked in most areas of health care as a Registered Nurse (RN), administrator, and supervisor for more than twenty-five years. She has observed common communication themes in each area she experienced. These themes adversely affected both patient and staff satisfaction, which resulted in increased operating costs, increased staff turnover, increased sick leave, and, in general, poor teamwork and lack of harmony. Melanie discovered that by shifting the communication patterns used, everything else shifted to create more positive outcomes for staff, patients, and administration.

Melanie lives in a cohousing community in Seattle, Washington.